The Ultimate Guide to Mediterranean Cuisine

Tasty and Healthy Recipes for the Eclectic Food Lover

By
Delia Bell

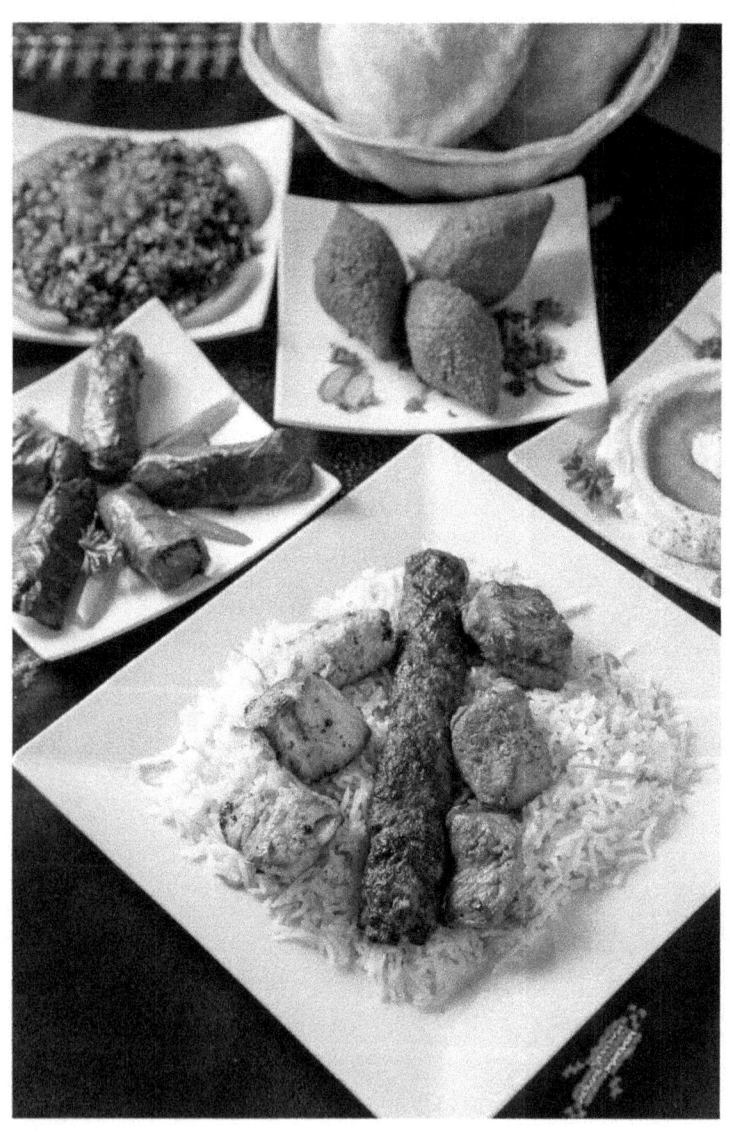

© Copyright 2021 by Delia Bell - All rights reserved.The following Book is reproduced below with the goal of providing information that is as accurate and reliable as possible. Regardless, purchasing this Book can be seen as consent to the fact that both the publisher and the author of this book are in no way experts on the topics discussed within and that any recommendations or suggestions that are made herein are for entertainment purposes only. Professionals should be consulted as needed prior to undertaking any of the action endorsed herein.

This declaration is deemed fair and valid by both the American Bar Association and the Committee of Publishers Association and is legally binding throughout the United States.

Furthermore, the transmission, duplication, or reproduction of any of the following work including specific information will be considered an illegal act irrespective of if it is done electronically or in print. This extends to creating a secondary or tertiary copy of the work or a recorded copy and is only allowed with the express written consent from the Publisher. All additional rights reserved.

The information in the following pages is broadly considered a truthful and accurate account of facts and as such, any inattention, use, or misuse of the information in question by the reader will render any resulting actions solely under their purview. There are no scenarios in which the publisher or the original author of this work can be in any fashion deemed liable for any hardship or damages that may befall them after undertaking information described herein.

Additionally, the information in the following pages is intended only for informational purposes and should thus be thought of as universal. As befitting its nature, it is presented without assurance regarding its prolonged validity or interim quality. Trademarks that are mentioned are done without written consent and can in no way be considered an endorsement from the trademark holder.

Table of Contents

INTRODUCTION   8
   What is the Mediterranean Diet?   8

Breakfast   14
   Cheesy Breakfast Pizza (cheese Manakish)   14
   Blueberries Quinoa   15
   Creamy Chorizo Bowls   17
   Mediterranean Omelet   18
   Hummus And Tomato Sandwich   20
   Sage Omelet   21
   Red Pepper And Artichoke Frittata   22
   Stuffed Figs   24
   Keto Egg Fast Snickerdoodle Crepes   25
   Cauliflower Hash Brown Breakfast Bowl   26
   Pumpkin Coconut Oatmeal   28
   Bacon, Vegetable And Parmesan Combo   29
   Mediterranean Crostini   30

Lunch & Dinner   32
   Chili Oregano Baked Cheese   32
   Mediterranean-style Vegetable Casserole   33
   Creamy Smoked Salmon Pasta   35
   Spiced Eggplant Stew   36
   Shrimp Soup   37
   Halloumi, Grape Tomato And Zucchini Skewers With Spinach-basil Oil   39
   Beef Bourguignon   41
   Mediterranean Flank Steak   43
   Spiced Grilled Flank Steak   44
   Pan Roasted Chicken With Olives And Lemon   45

Creamy Salmon Soup — 46

Salads & Side Dishes — **48**

Vinegar Cucumber Mix — 48
Crispy Fennel Salad — 49
Red Beet Feta Salad — 51
Cheese Potato Mash — 52
Provencal Summer Salad — 53
Sunflower Seeds And Arugula Garden Salad — 54
Pumpkin Mash — 55
Peppers Mix — 56
Lemony Carrots — 58
Roasted Vegetable Salad — 59
Chicken Kale Soup — 60
Mozzarella Pasta Mix — 61
Quinoa Salad — 63

Beans & Grains — **64**

Curried Chicken, Chickpeas And Raita Salad — 64
Bulgur Tomato Pilaf — 66
Garbanzo And Kidney Bean Salad — 67
Rice & Currant Salad Mediterranean Style — 69
Stuffed Tomatoes With Green Chili — 71
Red Wine Risotto — 74
Pasta Parmesan — 77
Orange, Dates And Asparagus On Quinoa Salad — 78
Tasty Lasagna Rolls — 80
Raisins, Nuts And Beef On Hashweh Rice — 82
Yangchow Chinese Style Fried Rice — 84
Cinnamon Quinoa Bars — 86
Cucumber Olive Rice — 87

Desserts **89**
    Soothing Red Smoothie 89
    Minty Orange Greek Yogurt 91
    Yogurt Mousse With Sour Cherry Sauce 92
    Vanilla Apple Pie 94
    Spinach Pancake Cake 95
    Fruit Salad With Orange Blossom Water 98
    Blueberry Frozen Yogurt 99
    Apple Pear Compote 101
    Cream Cheese Cake 103
    Nutmeg Lemon Pudding 105
    Yogurt Panna Cotta With Fresh Berries 106
    Flourless Chocolate Cake 107

INTRODUCTION

What is the Mediterranean Diet?

The Mediterranean diet is based on the diets of traditional eating habits from the 1960s of people from countries that surround the Mediterranean Sea, such as Greece, Italy, and Spain, and it encourages the consumption of fresh, seasonal, and local foods. The Mediterranean diet has become popular because individuals show low rates of heart disease, chronic disease, and obesity. The Mediterranean diet profile focuses on whole grains, good fats (fish, olive oil, nuts etc.), vegetables, fruits, fish, and very low consumption of any non-fish meat. Along with food, the Mediterranean diet emphasizes the need to spend time eating with family and physical activity. The Mediterranean diet is not a single prescribed diet, but rather a general food-based eating pattern, which is marked by local and cultural differences throughout the Mediterranean region.

The diet is generally characterized by a high intake of plant-based foods (e.g. fresh fruit and vegetables, nuts, and cereals) and olive oil, a moderate intake of fish and poultry, and low intakes of dairy products (mostly yoghurt and cheese), red and processed meats, and sweets. Wine is typically consumed in moderation and, normally, with a meal. A strong focus is placed on social and cultural aspects, such as communal mealtimes, resting after eating, and regular physical activity. Nowadays, however, the diet is no longer followed as widely as it was 30-50 years ago, as the diets of people living in these regions are becoming more 'Westernized' and higher in energy dense foods.

Benefits
The Mediterranean diet is not a weight loss, but increasing fiber intake and cutting out red meat, animal fats, and processed food may lead to weight loss. People who follow the diet may also have a lower risk of various diseases.

Heart health
In the 1950s, an American scientist, found that people living in the poorer areas of southern Italy had a lower risk of heart disease and death than those in wealthier parts of New York. Dr. Keys attributed this to diet. Since then, many studies have indicated that following a Mediterranean diet can help the body maintain healthy cholesterol levels and reduce the risk of high blood pressure and cardiovascular disease. The overall pattern of the Mediterranean diet is similar to their own dietary recommendations. A high proportion of calories on the diet come from fat, which can increase the risk of obesity. However, they also note that this fat is mainly unsaturated, which makes it a more healthful option than that from the typical American diet.

Protection from disease
The Mediterranean diet focuses on plant-based foods, and these are good sources of antioxidants.

The Mediterranean diet might offer protection from various cancers, and especially colorectal cancer. The reduction in risk may stem from the high intake of fruits, vegetables, and whole grains. By sticking to Mediterranean meals, people's levels of blood glucose and fats had decreased. During this time, there was also a lower incidence of stroke.

Diabetes
The Mediterranean diet may help prevent type 2 diabetes and improve markers of diabetes in people who already have the condition. Various other studies have concluded that following the Mediterranean diet can reduce the risk of type 2 diabetes and cardiovascular disease, which often occur together.

Food to eat
There is no single definition of the Mediterranean diet, but one group of scientists used the following as their 2015 basis of research.

Vegetables: Include 3 to 9 servings a day.

Fresh fruit: Up to 2 servings a day.

Cereals: Mostly whole grain from 1 to 13 servings a day.

Oil: Up to 8 servings of extra virgin (cold pressed) olive oil a day.

Fat — mostly unsaturated — made up 37% of the total calories. Unsaturated fat comes from plant sources, such as olives and avocado. The Mediterranean diet also provided 33 grams (g) of fiber a day. The baseline diet for this study provided around

2,200 calories a day. Typical ingredients. Here are some examples of ingredients that people often include in the Mediterranean diet.

Vegetables: Tomatoes, peppers, onions, eggplant, zucchini, cucumber, leafy green vegetables, plus others.
Fruits: Melon, apples, apricots, peaches, oranges, and lemons, and so on.
Legumes: Beans, lentils, and chickpeas.
Nuts and seeds: Almonds, walnuts, sunflower seeds, and cashews.
Unsaturated fat: Olive oil, sunflower oil, olives, and avocados.
Dairy products: Cheese and yogurt are the main dairy foods.
Cereals: These are mostly whole grain and include wheat and rice with bread accompanying many meals.
Fish: Sardines and other oily fish, as well as oysters and other shellfish. Poultry: Chicken or turkey.
Eggs: Chicken, quail, and duck eggs.
Drinks: A person can drink red wine in moderation.

The Mediterranean diet does not include strong liquor or carbonated and sweetened drinks. According to one definition, the diet limits red meat and sweets to less than 2 servings per week.

Food to avoid

Here's a list of foods you should generally limit while eating Mediterranean-style meals. Heavily processed foods. Let's be real: Many, many foods are processed to some degree. A can of beans has been processed, in the sense that the beans have been cooked before being canned. Olive oil has been processed, because olives have been turned into oil. But when we talk about limiting processed foods, this really means avoiding things like frozen meals with tons of sodium. You should also limit soda, desserts and candy. As the adage goes, if the ingredient list includes items that your great-grandparents wouldn't recognize as food, it's probably processed. If you're buying a packaged food that's as close to its whole-food form as possible — such as frozen fruit or veggies with nothing added — you're good to go.

Processed red meat

On the Mediterranean diet, you should minimize your intake of red meat, such as steak. What about processed red meat, such as hot dogs and bacon? You should avoid these foods or limit them as much as possible. A study published in BMJ found that regularly eating red meat, especially processed varieties, was associated with a higher risk of death. Butter. Here's another food that should be limited on the Mediterranean diet. Use olive oil instead, which has many heart health benefits and contains less saturated fat than butter. According to the USDA National Nutrient Database, butter has 7 grams of saturated fat per tablespoon, while olive oil has about 2 grams.

Refined grains

The Mediterranean diet is centered around whole grains, such as farro, millet, couscous and brown rice. With this eating style, you'll generally want to limit your intake of refined grains such as white pasta and white bread.

Alcohol

When you're following the Mediterranean diet, red wine should be your chosen alcoholic drink. This is because red wine offers health benefits, particularly for the heart. But it's important to limit intake of any type of alcohol to up to one drink per day for women, as well as men older than 65, and up to two drinks daily for men age 65 and younger. The amount that counts as a drink is 5 ounces of wine, 12 ounces of beer or 1.5 ounces of 80-proof liquor.

Breakfast

Cheesy Breakfast Pizza (cheese Manakish)

Servings: 1 Pizza
Cooking Time: 10 Minutes

Ingredients:
- 1 batch Multipurpose Dough
- 1/4 cup all-purpose flour
- 2 cups kashkaval cheese, grated
- 2 cups mozzarella cheese, grated

Directions:
1. Preheat the oven to 400°F. Flour a rolling pin and your counter.
2. Divide Multipurpose Dough into 6 equal portions, and roll out dough into 6- to 8-inch-diameter circles.
3. In a medium bowl, combine kashkaval cheese and mozzarella cheese. Divide cheese mixture into 6 portions, and sprinkle on each dough circle.
4. Place pizzas onto a baking sheet, and bake for 8 to 10 minutes or until cheese begins to bubble.
5. Remove pizzas from the oven, fold each pizza in half, and enjoy as is or with Yogurt Spread

Blueberries Quinoa

Servings: 4
Cooking Time: 0 Minutes

Ingredients:
- 2 cups almond milk
- 2 cups quinoa, already cooked
- ½ teaspoon cinnamon powder
- 1 tablespoon honey
- 1 cup blueberries
- ¼ cup walnuts, chopped

Directions:
1. In a bowl, mix the quinoa with the milk and the rest of the ingredients, toss, divide into smaller bowls and serve for breakfast.

Nutrition Info: calories 284, fat 14.3, fiber 3.2, carbs 15.4, protein 4.4

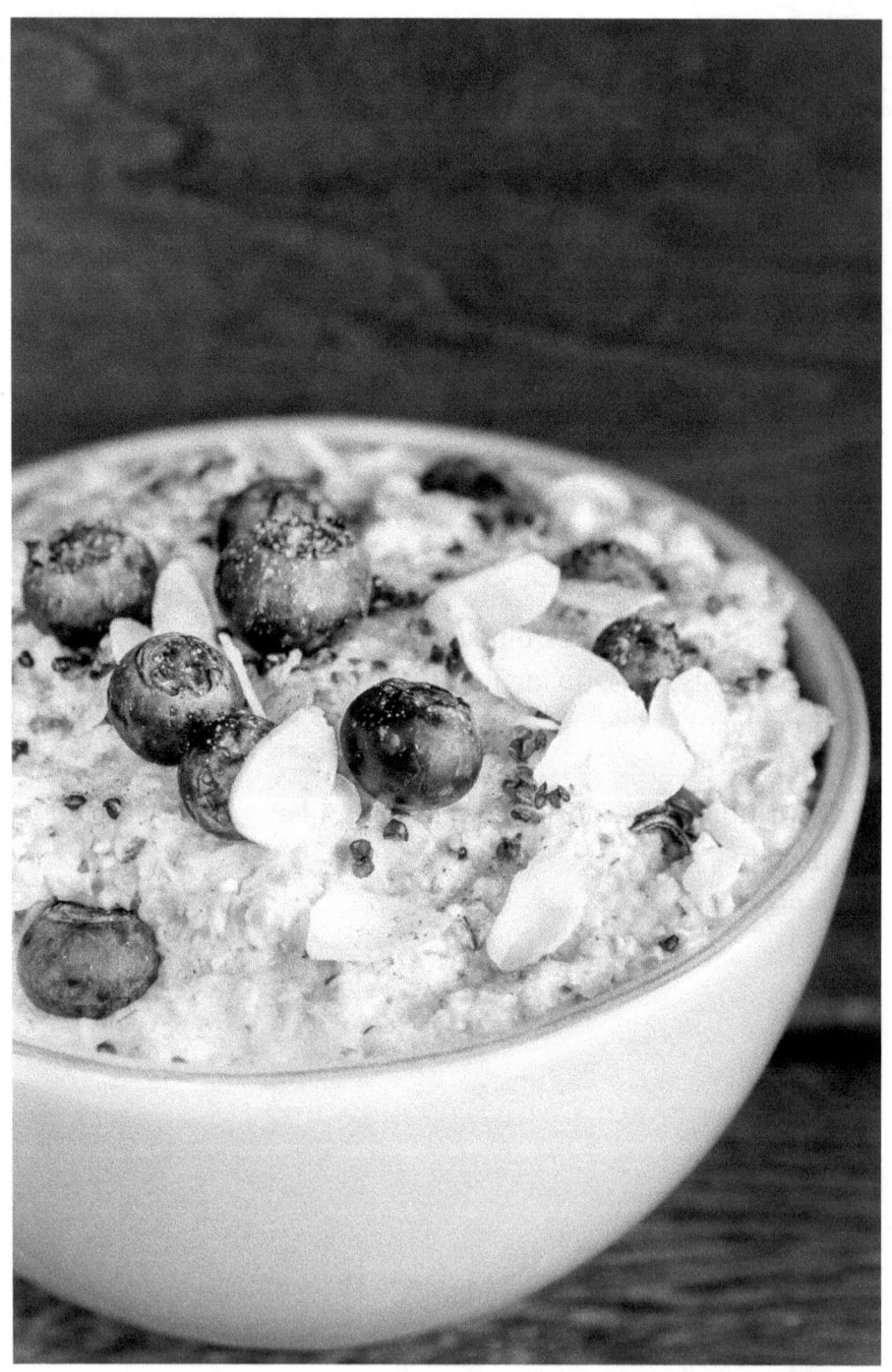

Creamy Chorizo Bowls

Servings: 4
Cooking Time: 15 Minutes

Ingredients:
- 9 oz chorizo
- 1 tablespoon almond butter
- ½ cup corn kernels
- 1 tomato, chopped
- ¾ cup heavy cream
- 1 teaspoon butter
- ¼ teaspoon chili pepper
- 1 tablespoon dill, chopped

Directions:
1. Chop the chorizo and place in the skillet.
2. Add almond butter and chili pepper.
3. Roast the chorizo for 3 minutes.
4. After this, add tomato and corn kernels.
5. Add butter and chopped dill. Mix up the mixture well. Cook for 2 minutes.
6. Close the lid and simmer the meal for 10 minutes over the low heat.
7. Transfer the cooked meal into the serving bowls.

Nutrition Info:Per Serving:calories 422, fat 36.2, fiber 1.2, carbs 7.3, protein 17.6

Mediterranean Omelet

Servings: 1 Omelet
Cooking Time: 10 Minutes

Ingredients:
- 2 TB. extra-virgin olive oil
- 2 TB. yellow onion, finely chopped
- 1 small clove garlic, minced
- 1/2 tsp. salt
- 1 cup fresh spinach, chopped
- 1/2 medium tomato, diced
- 2 large eggs
- 2 TB. whole or 2 percent milk
- 4 kalamata olives, pitted and chopped
- 1/2 tsp. ground black pepper
- 3 TB. crumbled feta cheese
- 1 TB. fresh parsley, finely chopped

Directions:
1. In a nonstick pan over medium heat, cook extra-virgin olive oil, yellow onion, and garlic for 3 minutes.
2. Add salt, spinach, and tomato, and cook for 4 minutes.
3. In a small bowl, whisk together eggs and whole milk.
4. Add kalamata olives and black pepper to the pan, and pour in eggs over sautéed vegetables.
5. Using a rubber spatula, slowly push down edges of eggs, letting raw egg form a new layer, and continue for about 2 minutes or until eggs are cooked.
6. Fold the omelet in half, and slide onto a plate. Top with feta cheese and fresh parsley, and serve warm.

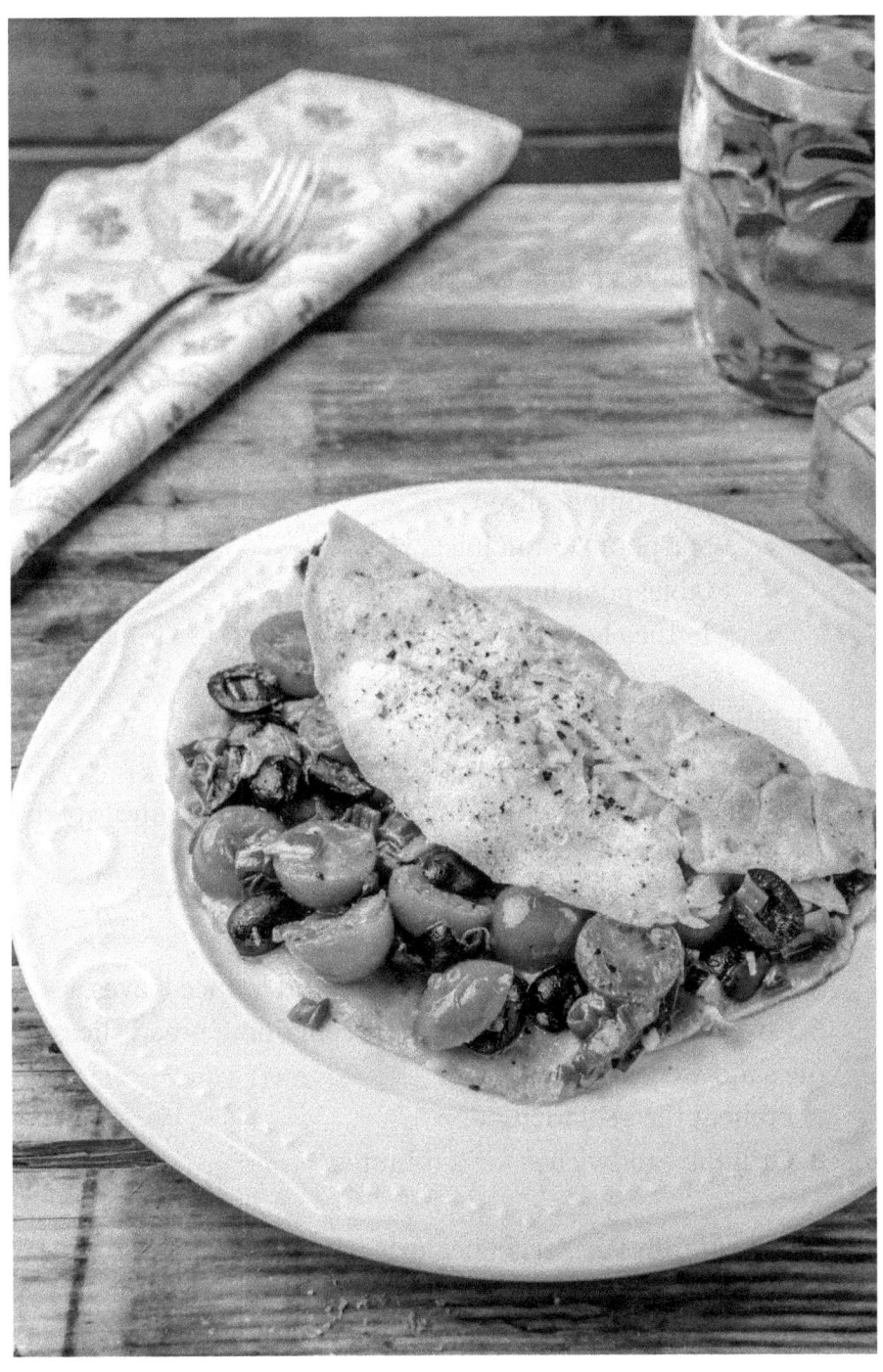

Hummus And Tomato Sandwich

Servings: 3
Cooking Time: 2 Minutes

Ingredients:
- 6 whole grain bread slices
- 1 tomato
- 3 Cheddar cheese slices
- ½ teaspoon dried oregano
- 1 teaspoon green chili paste
- ½ red onion, sliced
- 1 teaspoon lemon juice
- 1 tablespoon hummus
- 3 lettuce leaves

Directions:
1. Slice tomato into 6 slices.
2. In the shallow bowl mix up together dried oregano, green chili paste, lemon juice, and hummus.
3. Spread 3 bread slices with the chili paste mixture.
4. After this, place the sliced tomatoes on them.
5. Add sliced onion, Cheddar cheese, and lettuce leaves.
6. Cover the lettuce leaves with the remaining bread slices to get the sandwiches.
7. Preheat the grill to 365F.
8. Grill the sandwiches for 2 minutes.

Nutrition Info:Per Serving:calories 269, fat 12.1, fiber 5.1, carbs 29.6, protein 13.9

Sage Omelet

Servings: 8
Cooking Time: 25 Minutes

Ingredients:
- 8 eggs, beaten
- 6 oz Goat cheese, crumbled
- ½ teaspoon salt
- 3 tablespoons sour cream
- 1 teaspoon butter
- ½ teaspoon canola oil
- ¼ teaspoon sage
- ¼ teaspoon dried oregano
- 1 teaspoon chives, chopped

Directions:
1. Put butter in the skillet. Add canola oil and preheat the mixture until it is homogenous.
2. Meanwhile, in the mixing bowl combine together salt, sour cream, sage, dried oregano, and chives. Add eggs and stir the mixture carefully with the help of the spoon/fork.
3. Pour the egg mixture in the skillet with butter-oil liquid.
4. Sprinkle the omelet with goat cheese and close the lid.
5. Cook the breakfast for 20 minutes over the low heat. The cooked omelet should be solid.
6. Slice it into the servings and transfer in the plates.

Nutrition Info:Per Serving:calories 176, fat 13.7, fiber 0, carbs 0, protein 12.2

Red Pepper And Artichoke Frittata

Servings: 2
Cooking Time: 15 Minutes

Ingredients:
- 4 large eggs
- 1 can (14-ounce) artichoke hearts, rinsed, coarsely chopped
- 1 medium red bell pepper, diced
- 1 teaspoon dried oregano
- 1/4 cup Parmesan cheese, freshly grated
- 1/4 teaspoon red pepper, crushed
- 1/4 teaspoon salt, or to taste
- 2 garlic cloves, minced
- 2 teaspoons extra-virgin olive oil, divided
- Freshly ground pepper, to taste

Directions:
1. In a 10-inch non-stick skillet, heat 1 teaspoon of the olive oil over medium heat. Add the bell pepper; cook for about 2 minutes or until tender. Add the garlic and the red pepper; cook for about 30 seconds, stirring. Transfer the mixture to a plate and wipe the skillet clean.
2. In a medium mixing bowl, whisk the eggs. Stir in the artichokes, cheese, the bell pepper mixture, and season with salt and pepper.
3. Place an over rack 4 inches from the source of heat; preheat broiler.
4. Brush the skillet with the remaining 1 teaspoon olive oil and heat over medium heat. Pour the egg mixture into the skillet and tilt to evenly distribute. Reduce the heat to medium low; cook

for about 3-4 minutes, lifting the edges to allow the uncooked egg to flow underneath, until the bottom of the frittata is light golden.

5. Transfer the pan into the broiler, cook for about 1 1/2-2 1/2 minutes, or until the top is set.

6. Slide into a platter; cut into wedges and serve.

Nutrition Info:Per Serving:305 Cal, 18 g total fat (6 g sat. fat, 8 g mono), 432 mg chol., 734 mg sodium, 1639 mg pot., 18 g carb.,8 g fiber, 21 g protein.

Stuffed Figs

Servings: 2
Cooking Time: 15 Minutes

Ingredients:
- 7 oz fresh figs
- 1 tablespoon cream cheese
- ½ teaspoon walnuts, chopped
- 4 bacon slices
- ¼ teaspoon paprika
- ¼ teaspoon salt
- ½ teaspoon canola oil
- ½ teaspoon honey

Directions:
1. Make the crosswise cuts in every fig.
2. In the shallow bowl mix up together cream cheese, walnuts, paprika, and salt.
3. Fill the figs with cream cheese mixture and wrap in the bacon.
4. Secure the fruits with toothpicks and sprinkle with honey.
5. Line the baking tray with baking paper.
6. Place the prepared figs in the tray and sprinkle them with olive oil gently.
7. Bake the figs for 15 minutes at 350F.

Nutrition Info: Calories 299, fat 19.4, fiber 2.3, carbs 16.7, protein 15.2

Keto Egg Fast Snickerdoodle Crepes

Servings: 2
Cooking Time: 15 Minutes

Ingredients:
- 5 oz cream cheese, softened
- 6 eggs
- 1 teaspoon cinnamon
- Butter, for frying
- 1 tablespoon Swerve
- 2 tablespoons granulated Swerve
- 8 tablespoons butter, softened
- 1 tablespoon cinnamon

Directions:
1. For the crepes: Put all the ingredients together in a blender except the butter and process until smooth.
2. Heat butter on medium heat in a non-stick pan and pour some batter in the pan.
3. Cook for about 2 minutes, then flip and cook for 2 more minutes.
4. Repeat with the remaining mixture.
5. Mix Swerve, butter and cinnamon in a small bowl until combined.
6. Spread this mixture onto the centre of the crepe and serve rolled up.

Nutrition Info: Calories: 543 Carbs: 8g Fats: 51.6g Proteins: 15.7g Sodium: 455mg Sugar: 0.9g

Cauliflower Hash Brown Breakfast Bowl

Servings: 2
Cooking Time: 30 Minutes

Ingredients:
- 1 tablespoon lemon juice
- 1 egg
- 1 avocado
- 1 teaspoon garlic powder
- 2 tablespoons extra virgin olive oil
- 2 oz mushrooms, sliced
- ½ green onion, chopped
- ¼ cup salsa
- ¾ cup cauliflower rice
- ½ small handful baby spinach
- Salt and black pepper, to taste

Directions:
1. Mash together avocado, lemon juice, garlic powder, salt and black pepper in a small bowl.
2. Whisk eggs, salt and black pepper in a bowl and keep aside.
3. Heat half of olive oil over medium heat in a skillet and add mushrooms.
4. Sauté for about 3 minutes and season with garlic powder, salt, and pepper.
5. Sauté for about 2 minutes and dish out in a bowl.
6. Add rest of the olive oil and add cauliflower, garlic powder, salt and pepper.
7. Sauté for about 5 minutes and dish out.

8. Return the mushrooms to the skillet and add green onions and baby spinach.
9. Sauté for about 30 seconds and add whisked eggs.
10. Sauté for about 1 minute and scoop on the sautéed cauliflower hash browns.
11. Top with salsa and mashed avocado and serve.

Nutrition Info: Calories: 400 Carbs: 15.8g Fats: 36.7g Proteins: 8g Sodium: 288mg Sugar: 4.2g

Pumpkin Coconut Oatmeal

Servings: 6
Cooking Time: 13 Minutes

Ingredients:
- 2 cups oatmeal
- 1 cup of coconut milk
- 1 cup milk
- 1 teaspoon Pumpkin pie spices
- 2 tablespoons pumpkin puree
- 1 tablespoon Honey
- ½ teaspoon butter

Directions:
1. Pour coconut milk and milk in the saucepan. Add butter and bring the liquid to boil.
2. Add oatmeal, stir well with the help of a spoon and close the lid.
3. Simmer the oatmeal for 7 minutes over the medium heat.
4. Meanwhile, mix up together honey, pumpkin pie spices, and pumpkin puree.
5. When the oatmeal is cooked, add pumpkin puree mixture and stir well.
6. Transfer the cooked breakfast to the serving plates.

Nutrition Info:Per Serving:calories 232, fat 12.5, fiber 3.8, carbs 26.2, protein 5.9

Bacon, Vegetable And Parmesan Combo

Servings: 2
Cooking Time: 25 Minutes

Ingredients:
- 2 slices of bacon, thick-cut
- ½ tbsp mayonnaise
- ½ of medium green bell pepper, deseeded, chopped
- 1 scallion, chopped
- ¼ cup grated Parmesan cheese
- 1 tbsp olive oil

Directions:
1. Switch on the oven, then set its temperature to 375°F and let it preheat.
2. Meanwhile, take a baking dish, grease it with oil, and add slices of bacon in it.
3. Spread mayonnaise on top of the bacon, then top with bell peppers and scallions, sprinkle with Parmesan cheese and bake for about 25 minutes until cooked thoroughly.
4. When done, take out the baking dish and serve immediately.
5. For meal prepping, wrap bacon in a plastic sheet and refrigerate for up to 2 days.
6. When ready to eat, reheat bacon in the microwave and then serve.

Nutrition Info: Calories 197, Total Fat 13.8g, Total Carbs 4.7g, Protein 14.3g,
Sugar 1.9g, Sodium 662mg

Mediterranean Crostini

Servings: 4
Cooking Time: 15 Minutes

Ingredients:
- 12 slices (1/3-inch thick) whole-wheat baguette, toasted
- Coarse salt and freshly ground pepper
- For the spread:
- 1 can chickpeas (15 1/2 ounces), drained, rinsed
- 1/4 cup olive oil, extra-virgin
- 1 tablespoon lemon juice, freshly squeezed
- 1 small clove garlic, minced
- 2 tablespoons olive oil, extra-virgin, divided
- 2 tablespoons celery, finely diced, plus celery leaves for garnish 8 large green olives, pitted, cut into 1/8-inch slivers

Directions:
1. In a food processor, combine the spread ingredients and season with salt and pepper; set aside.
2. In a small mixing bowl, combine 1 tablespoon of olive oil and the remaining ingredients. Season with salt and pepper. Set aside.
3. Divide the spread between the toasted baguette slices, top with the relish. Drizzle the remaining1 tablespoon of olive oil over each and season with pepper. If desired, garnish with the celery leaves. Serve immediately.

Nutrition Info:Per Serving:603 Cal, 3.7 g total fat (3.7 g sat. fat), 0 mg chol., 781 mg sodium, 483 mg pot, 79.2 g carb.,9.6 g fiber,6.8 g sugar, 19.1 g protein.

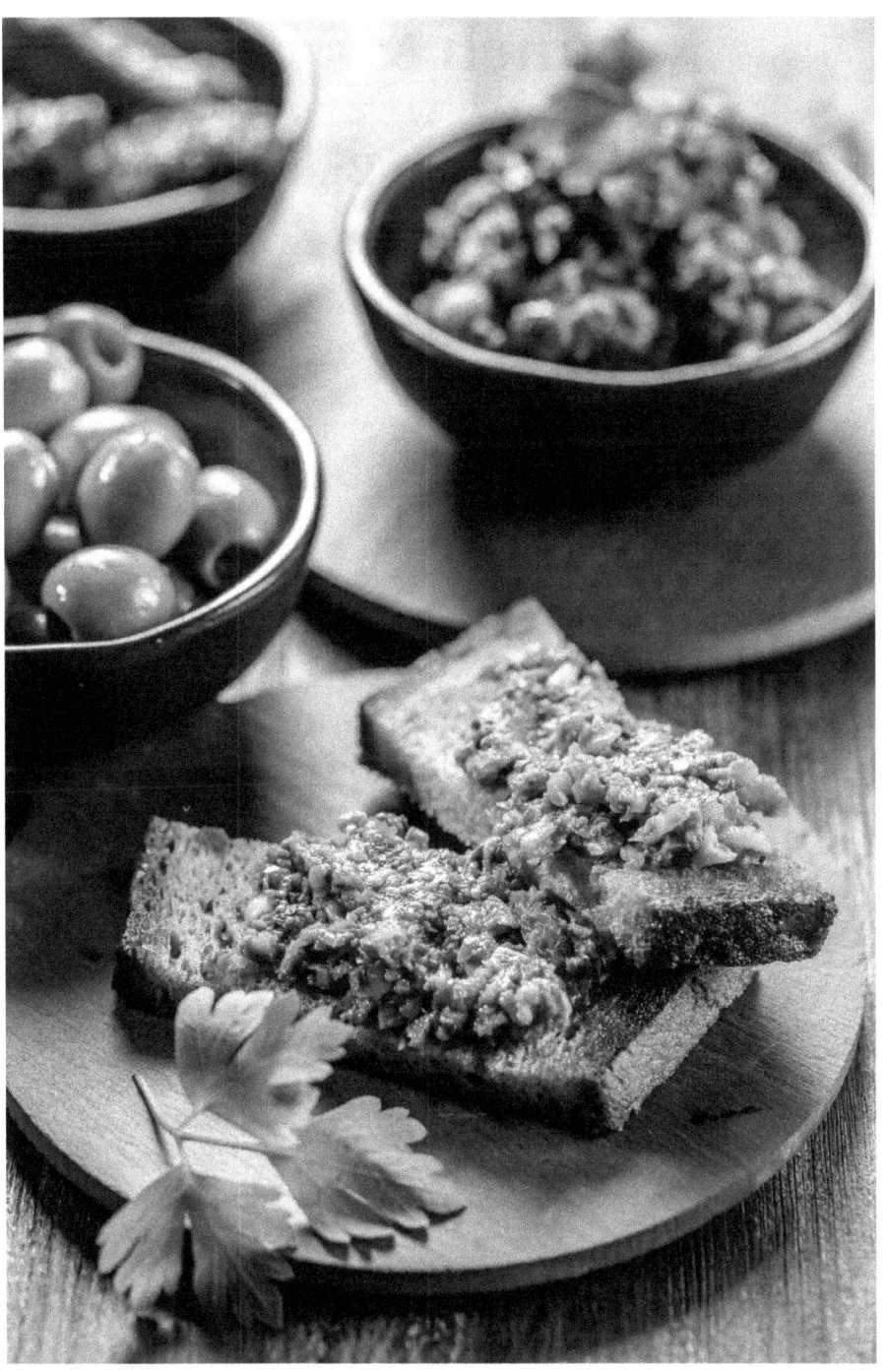

Lunch & Dinner

Chili Oregano Baked Cheese

Servings: 4
Cooking Time: 35 Minutes

Ingredients:
- 8 oz. feta cheese
- 4 oz. mozzarella, crumbled
- 1 chili pepper, sliced
- 1 teaspoon dried oregano
- 2 tablespoons olive oil

Directions:
1. Place the feta cheese in a small deep dish baking pan.
2. Top with the mozzarella then season with pepper slices and oregano.
3. Cover the pan with aluminum foil and cook in the preheated oven at 350F for 20 minutes.
4. Serve the cheese right away.

Nutrition Info: Per Serving:Calories:292 Fat:24.2g Protein:16.2g Carbohydrates:3.7g

Mediterranean-style Vegetable Casserole

Servings: 4
Cooking Time: 1 Hour

Ingredients:
- 1 aubergine or eggplant, sliced lengthwise
- 1 clove garlic, finely chopped
- 1 spring onion, very finely chopped
- 100 ml vegetable stock
- 2 courgettes or zucchini, sliced lengthwise
- 3 sprigs rosemary
- 4-5 tomatoes, sliced
- 5 tablespoons olive oil, divided
- 8 anchovy fillets, chopped
- 8 black olives

Directions:
1. Heat the oven to 325F.
2. In a greased oven-safe dish, layer the vegetables, adding the anchovies between each vegetable layer. Sprinkle the olives over the veggie layer, drizzle with 4 tablespoons of the olive oil, and then season with salt and pepper. Pour the stock; bake for 1 hour.
3. About 15 minutes before the end of baking, sprinkle the rosemary. When cooked, mix the green onion, garlic, and the remaining 1 tablespoon olive oil together; drizzle all over the baked veggies. Serve hot.

Nutrition Info:Per Serving:250 cal., 18 g total fat (2.5 g sat fat), <5 mg chol., 190 mg sodium, 980 mg potassium, 19 g carb., 7 g fiber, 11 g sugar, and 6 g protein.

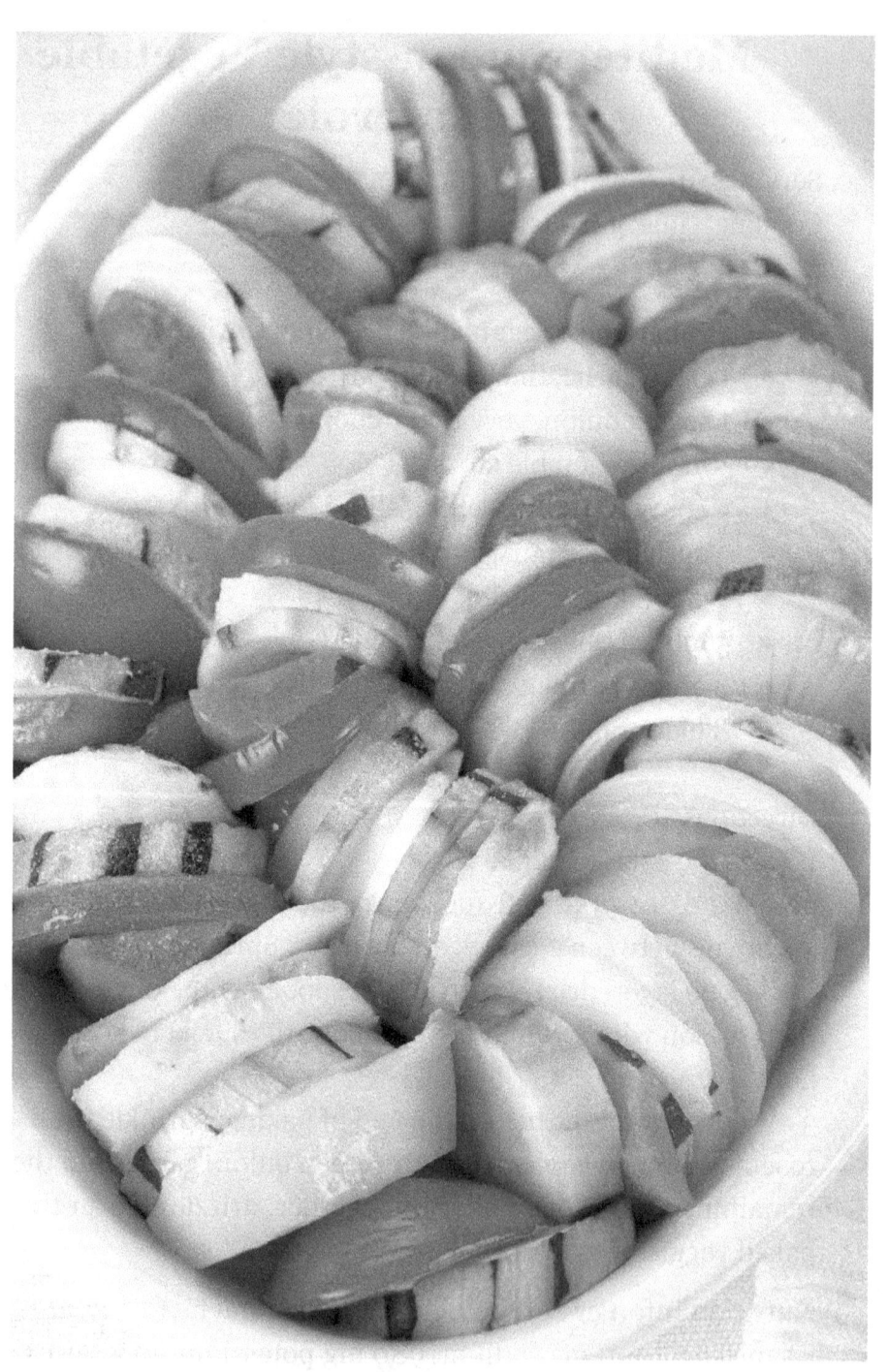

Creamy Smoked Salmon Pasta

Servings: 4
Cooking Time: 30 Minutes

Ingredients:
- 2 tablespoons olive oil
- 2 garlic cloves, chopped
- 1 shallot, chopped
- 4 oz. smoked salmon, chopped
- 1 cup green peas
- 1 cup heavy cream
- Salt and pepper to taste
- 1 pinch chili flakes
- 8 oz. penne

Directions:
1. Heat the oil in a skillet and add the garlic and shallot. Cook for 5 minutes until softened.
2. Add the salmon and peas, as well as salt and chili flakes.
3. Cook for 5 more minutes then add the cream.
4. Lower the heat and cook for 5 more minutes.
5. In the meantime, cook the penne in a large pot of water just until al dente.
6. Drain well then mix the pasta with the salmon sauce.
7. Serve the pasta fresh.

Nutrition Info: Per Serving:Calories:393 Fat:20.8g Protein:14.3g Carbohydrates:38.0g

Spiced Eggplant Stew

Servings: 4
Cooking Time: 45 Minutes

Ingredients:
- 4 eggplants, cubed
- Salt and black pepper to the taste
- 2 yellow onions, chopped
- 2 red bell peppers, chopped
- 30 ounces canned tomatoes, chopped
- 1 cup black olives, pitted and chopped
- ¼ teaspoon allspice, ground
- ½ teaspoon cinnamon powder
- 1 teaspoon oregano, dried
- A drizzle of olive oil
- A pinch of red chili flakes
- 3 tablespoons Greek yogurt

Directions:
1. Heat up a pot with the oil over medium high heat, add the onions, bell pepper, oregano, cinnamon and the allspice and sauté fro 5 minutes.
2. Add the rest of the ingredients except the flakes and the yogurt, bring to a simmer and cook over medium heat for 40 minutes.
3. Divide the stew into bowls, top each serving with the flakes and the yogurt and serve.

Nutrition Info: calories 256, fat 3.5, fiber 25.4, carbs 53.3, protein 8.8

Shrimp Soup

Servings: 6
Cooking Time: 5 Minutes

Ingredients:
- 1 cucumber, chopped
- 3 cups tomato juice
- 3 roasted red peppers, chopped
- 3 tablespoons olive oil
- 2 tablespoons balsamic vinegar
- 1 garlic clove, minced
- Salt and black pepper to the taste
- ½ teaspoon cumin, ground
- 1 pounds shrimp, peeled and deveined
- 1 teaspoon thyme, chopped

Directions:
1. In your blender, mix cucumber with tomato juice, red peppers, 2 tablespoons oil, the vinegar, cumin, salt, pepper and the garlic, pulse well, transfer to a bowl and keep in the fridge for 10 minutes.
2. Heat up a pot with the rest of the oil over medium heat, add the shrimp, salt, pepper and the thyme and cook for 2 minutes on each side.
3. Divide cold soup into bowls, top with the shrimp and serve.

Nutrition Info: calories 263, fat 11.1, fiber 2.4, carbs 12.5, protein 6.32

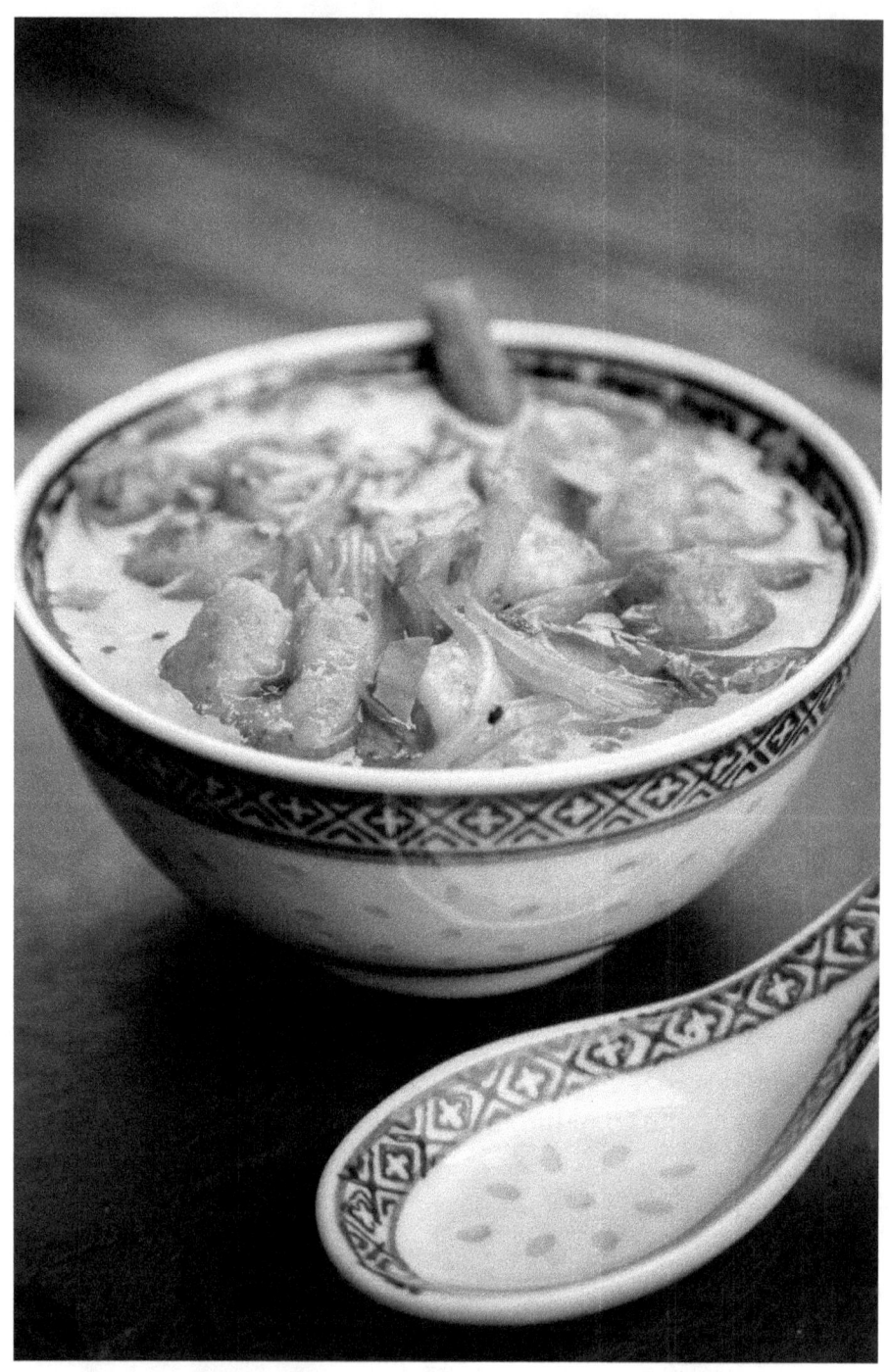

Halloumi, Grape Tomato And Zucchini Skewers With Spinach-basil Oil

Servings: 16
Cooking Time: 10 Minutes

Ingredients:
- 1 large zucchini, halved lengthways, cut into 8 pieces
- 16 grape tomatoes
- 180 g halloumi cheese, cut into 16 pieces
- Olive oil spray
- For the spinach-basil oil:
- 2 cups baby spinach leaves
- 2 cups fresh basil leaves
- 185 ml (3/4 cup) extra-virgin olive oil
- 125 ml (1/2 cup) light olive oil

Directions:
1. In a saucepan of boiling water, cook the spinach and the basil for about
30 seconds or until just wilted. Drain and cool under running cold water.
2. Place the cooked spinach and basil into a food processor. Add the light olive oil and the extra-virgin olive oil; process until the mixture is smooth. Transfer into an airtight container, refrigerate for 8 hours to develop the flavors.
3. Preheat the barbecue grill to medium-high.
4. Thread a piece of zucchini, halloumi cheese, and tomato into each skewer. Lightly spray with the olive oil spray.

5. Grill for about 4 minutes per side or until cooked through and golden brown.
6. Arrange the grilled skewers onto serving platter; serve immediately with the prepared spinach-basil oil.

Nutrition Info:Per Serving:192.2Cal, 20 g total fat (4 g sat. fat), 1 g carb., 1 g fiber, 1 g sugar, 3 g protein, and 328.8 mg sodium.

Beef Bourguignon

Servings: 8
Cooking Time: 2 Hours

Ingredients:
- 3 tablespoons olive oil
- 2 pounds beef roast, cubed
- 1 tablespoon all-purpose flour
- 3 sweet onions, chopped
- 2 carrots, sliced
- 4 garlic cloves, minced
- 1 chili pepper, sliced
- 1 pound button mushrooms
- 1 ½ cups beef stock
- ½ cup dark beer
- 2 bay leaves
- 1 thyme sprig
- 1 rosemary sprig
- Salt and pepper to taste

Directions:
1. Sprinkle the beef with flour.
2. Heat the oil in a deep heavy pot and add the beef roast.
3. Cook on all sides for 5 minutes or until browned.
4. Add the onions, carrots and chili and cook for 5 more minutes.
5. Add the mushrooms, stock, beer, bay leaves, thyme, rosemary, salt and pepper.
6. Cover the pot and cook on low heat for 1 ½ hours.
7. Serve the stew warm and fresh.

Nutrition Info: Per Serving:Calories:306 Fat:12.6g Protein:37.6g Carbohydrates:9.0g

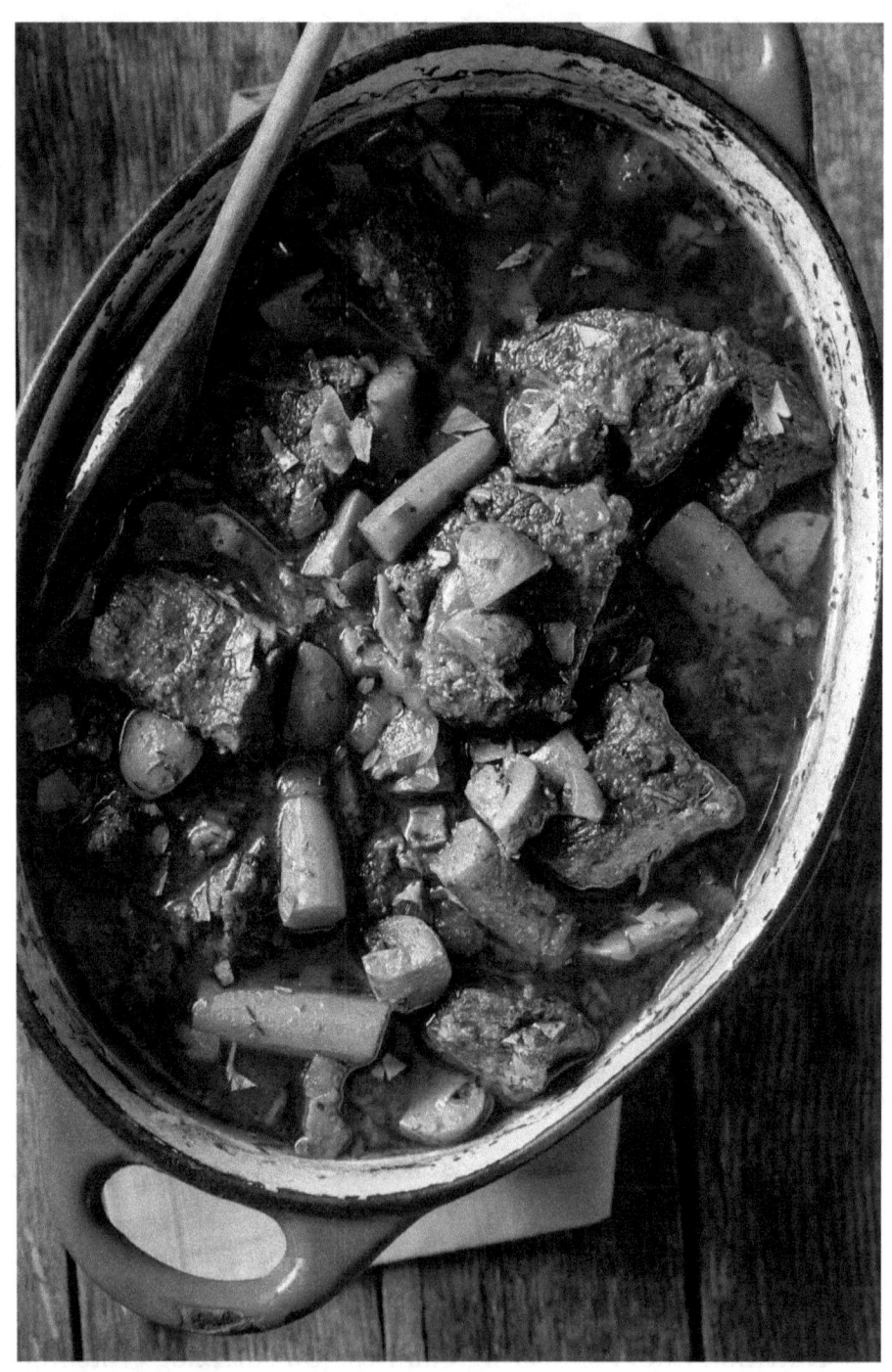

Mediterranean Flank Steak

Servings: 4
Cooking Time: 40 Minutes

Ingredients:
- 4 flank steaks
- 1 lemon, juiced
- 1 orange, juiced
- 4 garlic cloves, chopped
- 1 teaspoon Dijon mustard
- 1 teaspoon chopped thyme
- 1 teaspoon dried sage
- 2 tablespoons olive oil
- Salt and pepper to taste

Directions:
1. Combine the flank steaks and the rest of the ingredients in a zip lock bag.
2. Refrigerate for 30 minutes.
3. Heat a grill pan over medium flame and place the steaks on the grill.
4. Cook on each side for 6-7 minutes.
5. Serve the steaks warm and fresh.

Nutrition Info: Per Serving:Calories:234 Fat:13.4g Protein:21.6g Carbohydrates:6.7g

Spiced Grilled Flank Steak

Servings: 4
Cooking Time: 40 Minutes

Ingredients:
- 4 flank steaks
- 1 teaspoon chili powder
- 1 teaspoon ground coriander
- 1 teaspoon ground cumin
- 1 teaspoon mustard powder
- Salt and pepper to taste

Directions:
1. Season the steaks with salt and pepper then sprinkle with chili, coriander, cumin and mustard powder.
2. Allow to rest for 20 minutes then heat a grill pan over medium flame and place the steaks on the grill.
3. Cook on each side for 5-7 minutes and serve the steaks warm and fresh.

Nutrition Info: Per Serving:Calories:202 Fat:8.8g Protein:28.2g Carbohydrates:0.9g

Pan Roasted Chicken With Olives And Lemon

Servings: 4
Cooking Time: 50 Minutes

Ingredients:
- 4 chicken legs
- Salt and pepper to taste
- 3 tablespoons olive oil
- 1 lemon, juiced
- 1 orange, juiced
- 1 jalapeno, sliced
- 2 garlic cloves, chopped
- ½ cup green olives, sliced
- ¼ cup black olives, pitted and sliced
- 1 thyme sprig
- 1 rosemary sprig

Directions:
1. Season the chicken with salt and pepper.
2. Heat the oil in a skillet and add the chicken.
3. Cook on each side for 5 minutes until golden brown then add the rest of the ingredients and continue cooking on medium heat for15 minutes.
4. Serve the chicken and the sauce warm.

Nutrition Info: Per Serving:Calories:319 Fat:18.9g Protein:29.7g Carbohydrates:8.0g

Creamy Salmon Soup

Servings: 6
Cooking Time: 15 Minutes

Ingredients:
- 2 tablespoon olive oil
- 1 red onion, chopped
- Salt and white pepper to the taste
- 3 gold potatoes, peeled and cubed
- 2 carrots, chopped
- 4 cups fish stock
- 4 ounces salmon fillets, boneless and cubed
- ½ cup heavy cream
- 1 tablespoon dill, chopped

Directions:
1. Heat up a pan with the oil over medium heat, add the onion, and sauté for 5 minutes.
2. Add the rest of the ingredients expect the cream, salmon and the dill, bring to a simmer and cook for 5-6 minutes more.
3. Add the salmon, cream and the dill, simmer for 5 minutes more, divide into bowls and serve.

Nutrition Info: calories 214, fat 16.3, fiber 1.5, carbs 6.4, protein 11.8

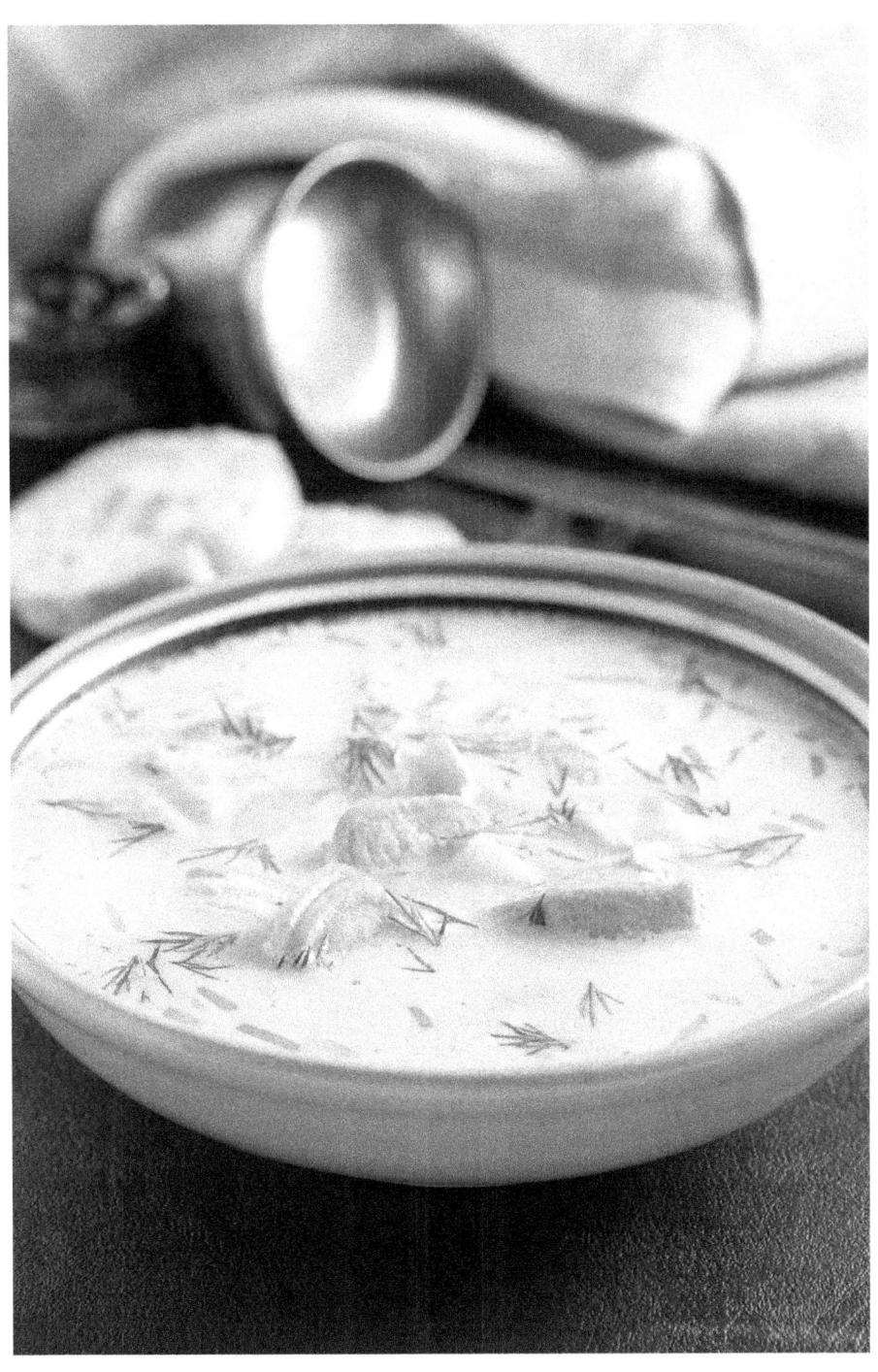

Salads & Side Dishes

Vinegar Cucumber Mix

Servings: 6
Cooking Time: 0 Minutes

Ingredients:
- 1 tablespoon olive oil
- 4 cucumbers, sliced
- Salt and black pepper to the taste
- 1 red onion, chopped
- 3 tablespoons red wine vinegar
- 1 bunch basil, chopped
- 1 teaspoon honey

Directions:
1. In a bowl, mix the vinegar with the basil, salt, pepper, the oil and the honey and whisk well.
2. In a bowl, mix the cucumber with the onion and the vinaigrette, toss and serve as a side salad.

Nutrition Info: calories 182, fat 7.8, fiber 2.1, carbs 4.3, protein 4.1

Crispy Fennel Salad

Servings: 2
Cooking Time: 15 Minutes

Ingredients:
- 1 fennel bulb, finely sliced
- 1 grapefruit, cut into segments
- 1 orange, cut into segments
- 2 tablespoons almond slices, toasted
- 1 teaspoon chopped mint
- 1 tablespoon chopped dill
- Salt and pepper to taste
- 1 tablespoon grape seed oil

Directions:
1. Mix the fennel bulb with the grapefruit and orange segments on a platter.
2. Top with almond slices, mint and dill then drizzle with the oil and season with salt and pepper.
3. Serve the salad as fresh as possible.

Nutrition Info: Per Serving:Calories:104 Fat:0.5g Protein:3.1g Carbohydrates:25.5g

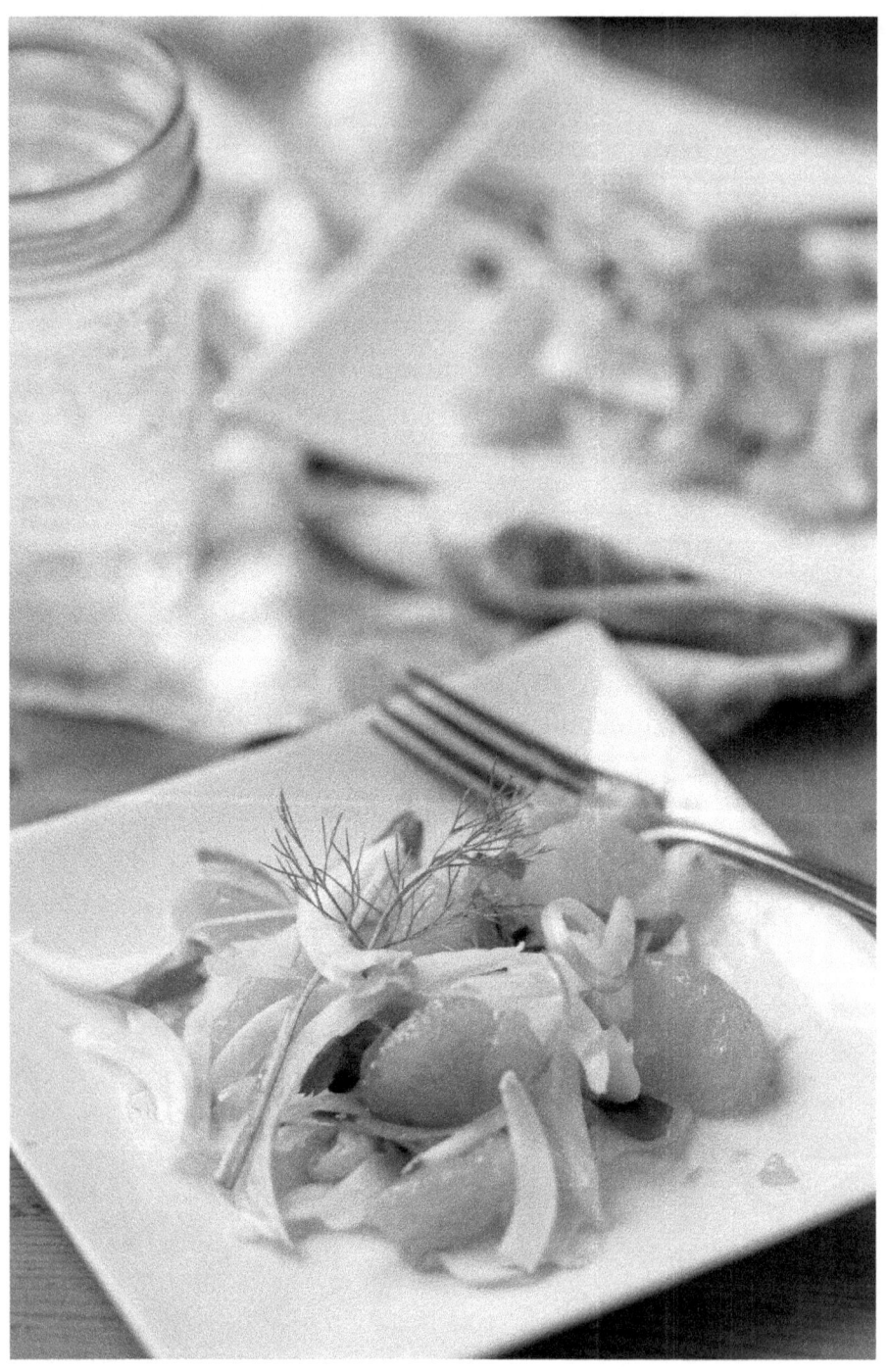

Red Beet Feta Salad

Servings: 4
Cooking Time: 15 Minutes

Ingredients:
- 6 red beets, cooked and peeled
- 3 oz. feta cheese, cubed
- 2 tablespoons extra virgin olive oil
- 2 tablespoons balsamic vinegar

Directions:
1. Combine the beets and feta cheese on a platter.
2. Drizzle with oil and vinegar and serve right away.

Nutrition Info: Per Serving:Calories: 230 Fat: 12.0g Protein: 7.3g Carbohydrates: 26.3g

Cheese Potato Mash

Servings: 8
Cooking Time: 20 Minutes

Ingredients:
- 2 pounds gold potatoes, peeled and cubed
- 1 and ½ cup cream cheese, soft
- Sea salt and black pepper to the taste
- ½ cup almond milk
- 2 tablespoons chives, chopped

Directions:
1. Put potatoes in a pot, add water to cover, add a pinch of salt, bring to a simmer over medium heat, cook for 20 minutes, drain and mash them.
2. Add the rest of the ingredients except the chives and whisk well.
3. Add the chives, stir, divide between plates and serve as a side dish.

Nutrition Info: calories 243, fat 14.2, fiber 1.4, carbs 3.5, protein 1.4

Provencal Summer Salad

Servings: 4
Cooking Time: 25 Minutes

Ingredients:
- 1 zucchini, sliced
- 1 eggplant, sliced
- 2 red onions, sliced
- 2 tomatoes, sliced
- 1 teaspoon dried mint
- 2 garlic cloves, minced
- 2 tablespoons balsamic vinegar
- Salt and pepper to taste

Directions:
1. Season the zucchini, eggplant, onions and tomatoes with salt and pepper. Cook the vegetable slices on the grill until browned.
2. Transfer the vegetables in a salad bowl then add the mint, garlic and vinegar.
3. Serve the salad right away.

Nutrition Info: Per Serving:Calories: 74 Fat: 0.5g Protein: 3.0g Carbohydrates: 16.5g

Sunflower Seeds And Arugula Garden Salad

Servings: 6
Cooking Time: 0 Minutes

Ingredients:
- ¼ tsp black pepper
- ¼ tsp salt
- 1 tsp fresh thyme, chopped
- 2 tbsp sunflower seeds, toasted
- 2 cups red grapes, halved
- 7 cups baby arugula, loosely packed
- 1 tbsp coconut oil
- 2 tsp honey
- 3 tbsp red wine vinegar
- ½ tsp stone-ground mustard

Directions:
1. In a small bowl, whisk together mustard, honey and vinegar. Slowly pour oil as you whisk.
2. In a large salad bowl, mix thyme, seeds, grapes and arugula.
3. Drizzle with dressing and serve.

Nutrition Info: Calories per serving: 86.7; Protein: 1.6g; Carbs: 13.1g; Fat: 3.1g 707. Ginger

Pumpkin Mash

Servings: 4
Cooking Time: 30 Minutes

Ingredients:
- 10 oz pumpkin, peeled
- ½ teaspoon butter
- ¾ teaspoon ground ginger
- 1/3 teaspoon salt

Directions:
1. Chop the pumpkin into cubes and bake in the preheated 360F oven for 30 minutes or until the pumpkin is soft.
2. After this, transfer the pumpkin cubes in the food processor.
3. Add butter, salt, and ground ginger.
4. Blend the vegetable until you get puree or use the potato masher for this step.

Nutrition Info:Per Serving:calories 30, fat 0.7, fiber 2.1, carbs 6, protein 0.8 708. Yogurt

Peppers Mix

Servings: 4
Cooking Time: 15 Minutes

Ingredients:
- 2 red bell peppers, cut into thick strips
- 2 tablespoons olive oil
- 3 shallots, chopped
- 3 garlic cloves, minced
- Salt and black pepper to the taste
- ½ cup Greek yogurt
- 1 tablespoon cilantro, chopped

Directions:
1. Heat up a pan with the oil over medium heat, add the shallots and garlic, stir and cook for 5 minutes.
2. Add the rest of the ingredients, toss, cook for 10 minutes more, divide the mix between plates and serve as a side dish.

Nutrition Info: calories 274, fat 11, fiber 3.5, protein 13.3, carbs 6.5

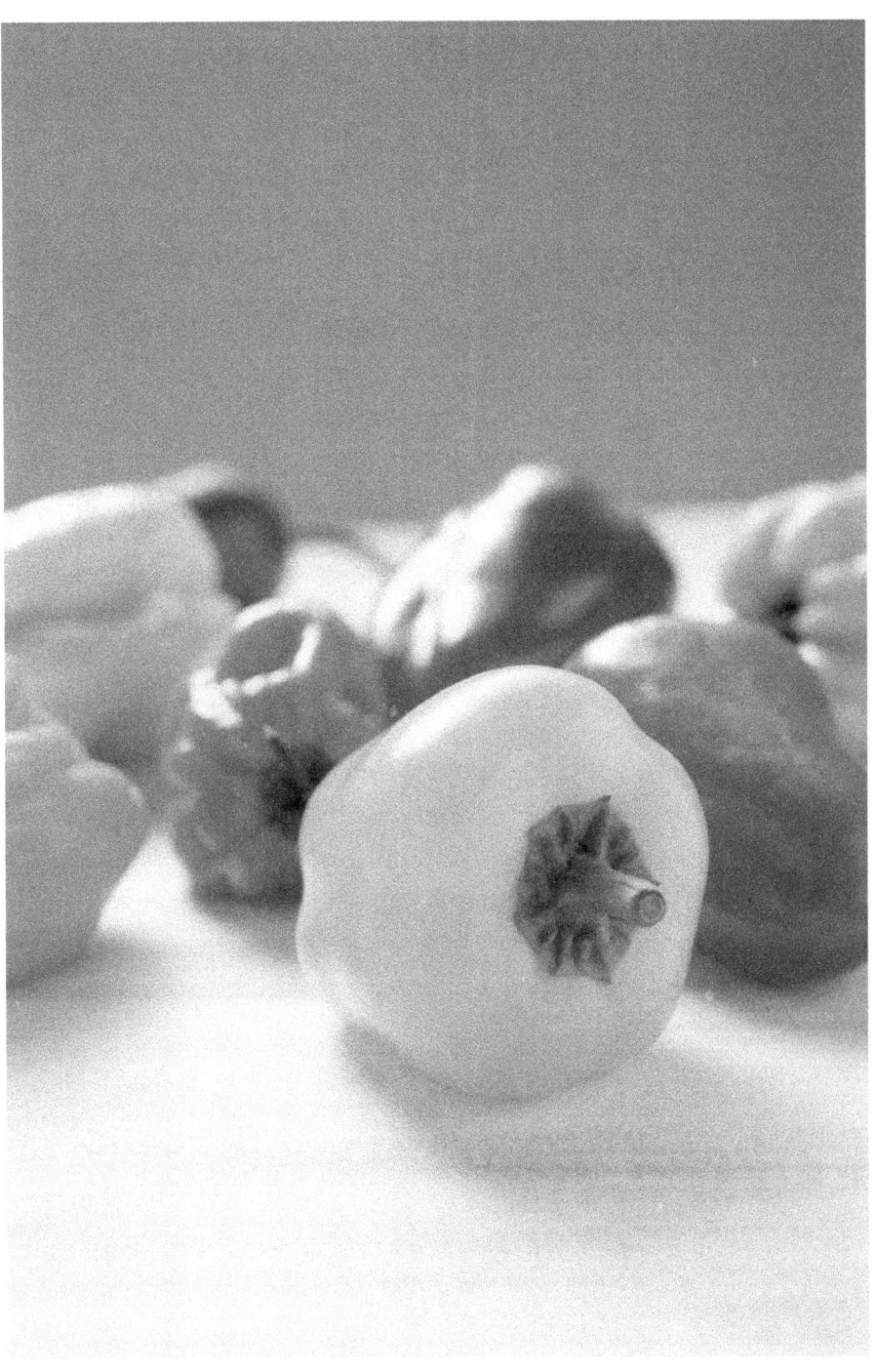

Lemony Carrots

Servings: 4
Cooking Time: 40 Minutes

Ingredients:
- 3 tablespoons olive oil
- 2 pounds baby carrots, trimmed
- Salt and black pepper to the taste
- ½ teaspoon lemon zest, grated
- 1 tablespoon lemon juice
- 1/3 cup Greek yogurt
- 1 garlic clove, minced
- 1 teaspoon cumin, ground
- 1 tablespoon dill, chopped

Directions:
1. In a roasting pan, combine the carrots with the oil, salt, pepper and the rest of the ingredients except the dill, toss and bake at 400 degrees F for 20 minutes.
2. Reduce the temperature to 375 degrees F and cook for 20 minutes more.
3. Divide the mix between plates, sprinkle the dill on top and serve.

Nutrition Info: calories 192, fat 5.4, fiber 3.4, carbs 7.3, protein 5.6

Roasted Vegetable Salad

Servings: 6
Cooking Time: 30 Minutes

Ingredients:
- ½ pound baby carrots
- 2 red onions, sliced
- 1 zucchini, sliced
- 2 eggplants, cubed
- 1 cauliflower, cut into florets
- 1 sweet potato, peeled and cubed
- 1 endive, sliced
- 3 tablespoons extra virgin olive oil
- 1 teaspoon dried basil
- Salt and pepper to taste
- 1 lemon, juiced
- 1 tablespoon balsamic vinegar

Directions:
1. Combine the vegetables with the oil, basil, salt and pepper in a deep dish baking pan and cook in the preheated oven at 350F for 25-30 minutes.
2. When done, transfer in a salad bowl and add the lemon juice and vinegar.
3. Serve the salad fresh.

Nutrition Info: Per Serving:Calories:164 Fat:7.6g Protein:3.7g Carbohydrates:24.2g

Chicken Kale Soup

Servings: 6
Cooking Time: 6 Hours 10 Minutes

Ingredients:
- 2 pounds chicken breast, skinless
- ⅓ cuponation
- 1tablespoonolive oil
- 14ounceschicken bone broth
- ½ cup olive oil
- 4 cups chicken stock
- ¼ cup lemon juice
- 5 ounces baby kale leaves
- Salt, to taste

Directions:
1. Season chicken with salt and black pepper.
2. Heat olive oil over medium heat in a large skillet and add seasoned chicken.
3. Reduce the temperature and cook for about 15 minutes.
4. Shred the chicken and place in the crock pot.
5. Process the chicken broth and onions in a blender and blend until smooth.
6. Pour into crock pot and stir in the remaining ingredients.
7. Cook on low for about 6 hours, stirring once while cooking.

Nutrition Info: Calories: 261 Carbs: 2g Fats: 21g Proteins: 14.1g Sodium: 264mg Sugar: 0.3g

Mozzarella Pasta Mix

Servings: 2
Cooking Time: 15 Minutes

Ingredients:
- 2 oz whole grain elbow macaroni
- 1 tablespoon fresh basil
- ¼ cup cherry size Mozzarella
- ½ cup cherry tomatoes, halved
- 1 tablespoon olive oil
- 1 teaspoon dried marjoram
- 1 cup water, for cooking

Directions:
1. Boil elbow macaroni in water for 15 minutes. Drain water and chill
macaroni a little.
2. Chop fresh basil roughly and place it in the salad bowl.
3. Add Mozzarella, cherry tomatoes, dried marjoram, olive oil, and macaroni.
4. Mix up salad well.

Nutrition Info:Per Serving:calories 170, fat 9.7, fiber 1.1, carbs 15, protein 6

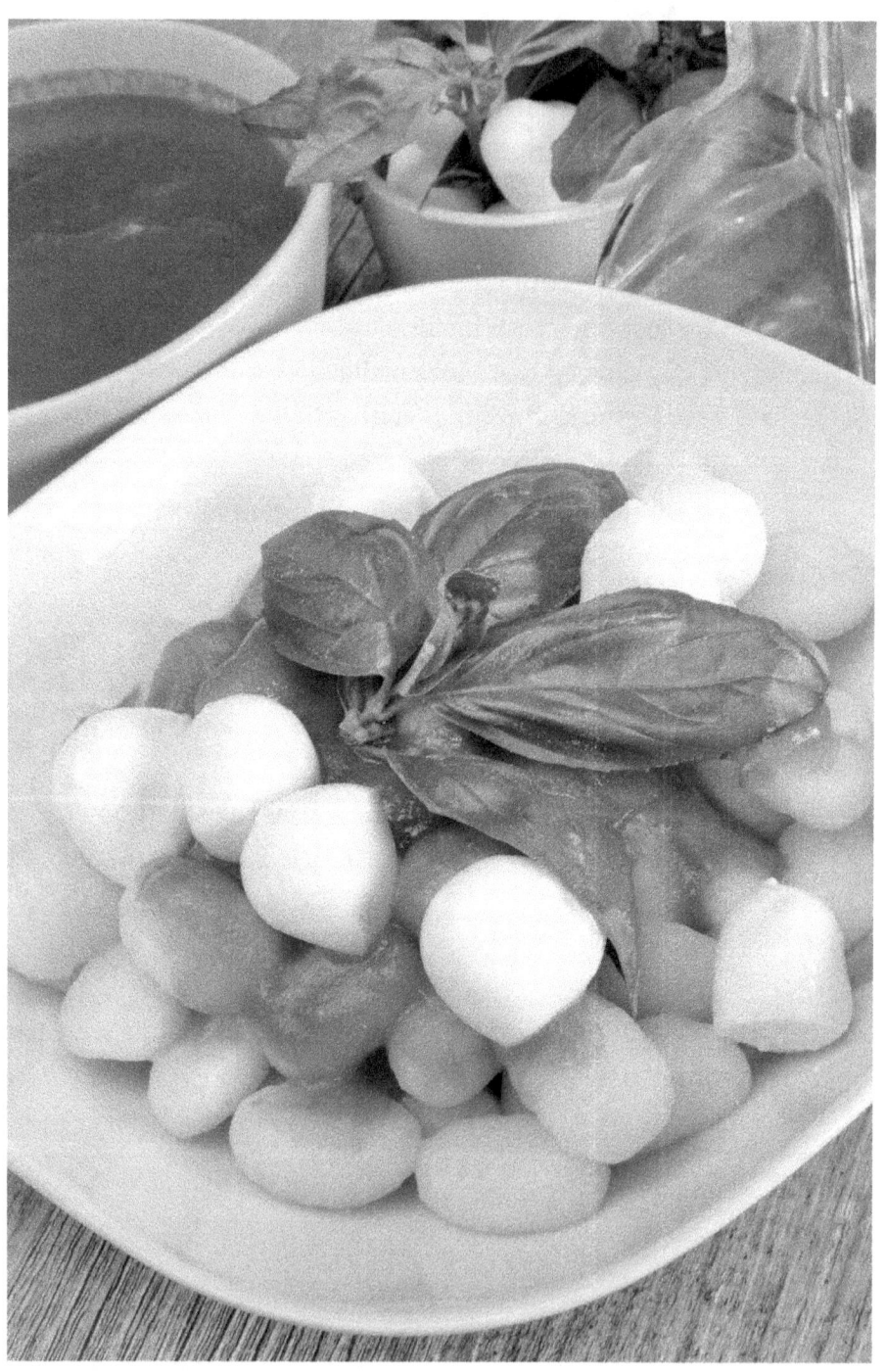

Quinoa Salad

Servings: 2 Cups
Cooking Time: 20 Minutes

Ingredients:
- 2 cups red quinoa
- 4 cups water
- 1 (15-oz.) can chickpeas, drained
- 1 medium red onion, chopped (1/2 cup)
- 3 TB. fresh mint leaves, finely chopped
- 1/4 cup extra-virgin olive oil
- 3 TB. fresh lemon juice
- 1/2 tsp. salt
- 1/2 tsp. fresh ground black pepper

Directions:
1. In a medium saucepan over medium-high heat, bring red quinoa and water to a boil. Cover, reduce heat to low, and cook for 20 minutes or until water is absorbed and quinoa is tender. Let cool.
2. In a large bowl, add quinoa, chickpeas, red onion, and mint.
3. In a small bowl, whisk together extra-virgin olive oil, lemon juice, salt, and black pepper.
4. Pour dressing over quinoa mixture, and stir well to combine.
5. Serve immediately, or refrigerate and enjoy for up to 2 or 3 days.

Beans & Grains

Curried Chicken, Chickpeas And Raita Salad

Servings: 8
Cooking Time: 15 Minutes

Ingredients:
- 1 cup red grapes, halved
- 3-4 cups rotisserie chicken, meat coarsely shredded
- 2 tbsp cilantro
- 1 cup plain yogurt
- 2 medium tomatoes, chopped
- 1 tsp ground cumin
- 1 tbsp curry powder
- 2 tbsp olive oil
- 1 tbsp minced peeled ginger
- 1 tbsp minced garlic
- 1 medium onion, chopped
- ¼ tsp cayenne
- ½ tsp turmeric
- 1 tsp ground cumin
- 1 19-oz can chickpeas, rinsed, drained and patted dry
- 1 tbsp olive oil
- ½ cup sliced and toasted almonds
- 2 tbsp chopped mint
- 2 cups cucumber, peeled, cored and chopped
- 1 cup plain yogurt

Directions:
1. To make the chicken salad, on medium low fire, place a medium nonstick saucepan and heat oil.
2. Sauté ginger, garlic and onion for 5 minutes or until softened while stirring occasionally.
3. Add 1 ½ tsp salt, cumin and curry. Sauté for two minutes.
4. Increase fire to medium high and add tomatoes. Stirring frequently, cook for 5 minutes.
5. Pour sauce into a bowl, mix in chicken, cilantro and yogurt. Stir to combine and let it stand to cool to room temperature.
6. To make the chickpeas, on a nonstick fry pan, heat oil for 3 minutes.
7. Add chickpeas and cook for a minute while stirring frequently.
8. Add ¼ tsp salt, cayenne, turmeric and cumin. Stir to mix well and cook for two minutes or until sauce is dried.
9. Transfer to a bowl and let it cool to room temperature.
10. To make the raita, mix ½ tsp salt, mint, cucumber and yogurt. Stir thoroughly to combine and dissolve salt.
11. To assemble, in four 16-oz lidded jars or bowls layer the following: curried chicken, raita, chickpeas and garnish with almonds.
12. You can make this recipe one day ahead and refrigerate for 6 hours before serving.

Nutrition Info: Calories per serving: 381; Protein: 36.1g; Carbs: 27.4g; Fat: 15.5g

Bulgur Tomato Pilaf

Servings: 1 Cup
Cooking Time: 27 Minutes

Ingredients:
- 1 lb. ground beef
- 3 TB. extra-virgin olive oil
- 1 large yellow onion, finely chopped
- 2 medium tomatoes, diced
- 11/2 tsp. salt
- 1 tsp. ground black pepper
- 2 cups plain tomato sauce
- 2 cups water
- 2 cups bulgur wheat, grind #2

Directions:
1. In a large, 3-quart pot over medium heat, brown beef for 5 minutes, breaking up chunks with a wooden spoon.
2. Add extra-virgin olive oil and yellow onion, and cook for 5 minutes.
3. Stir in tomatoes, salt, and black pepper, and cook for 5 minutes.
4. Add tomato sauce and water, and simmer for 10 minutes.
5. Add bulgur wheat, and cook for 2 minutes. Remove from heat, cover, and let sit for 5 minutes. Uncover, fluff bulgur with a fork, cover, and let sit for 5 more minutes.
6. Serve warm.

Garbanzo And Kidney Bean Salad

Servings: 4
Cooking Time: 0 Minutes

Ingredients:
- 1 (15 ounce) can kidney beans, drained
- 1 (15.5 ounce) can garbanzo beans, drained
- 1 lemon, zested and juiced
- 1 medium tomato, chopped
- 1 teaspoon capers, rinsed and drained
- 1/2 cup chopped fresh parsley
- 1/2 teaspoon salt, or to taste
- 1/4 cup chopped red onion
- 3 tablespoons extra virgin olive oil

Directions:
1. In a salad bowl, whisk well lemon juice, olive oil and salt until dissolved.
2. Stir in garbanzo, kidney beans, tomato, red onion, parsley, and capers. Toss well to coat.
3. Allow flavors to mix for 30 minutes by setting in the fridge.
4. Mix again before serving.

Nutrition Info: Calories per serving: 329; Protein: 12.1g; Carbs: 46.6g; Fat: 12.0g

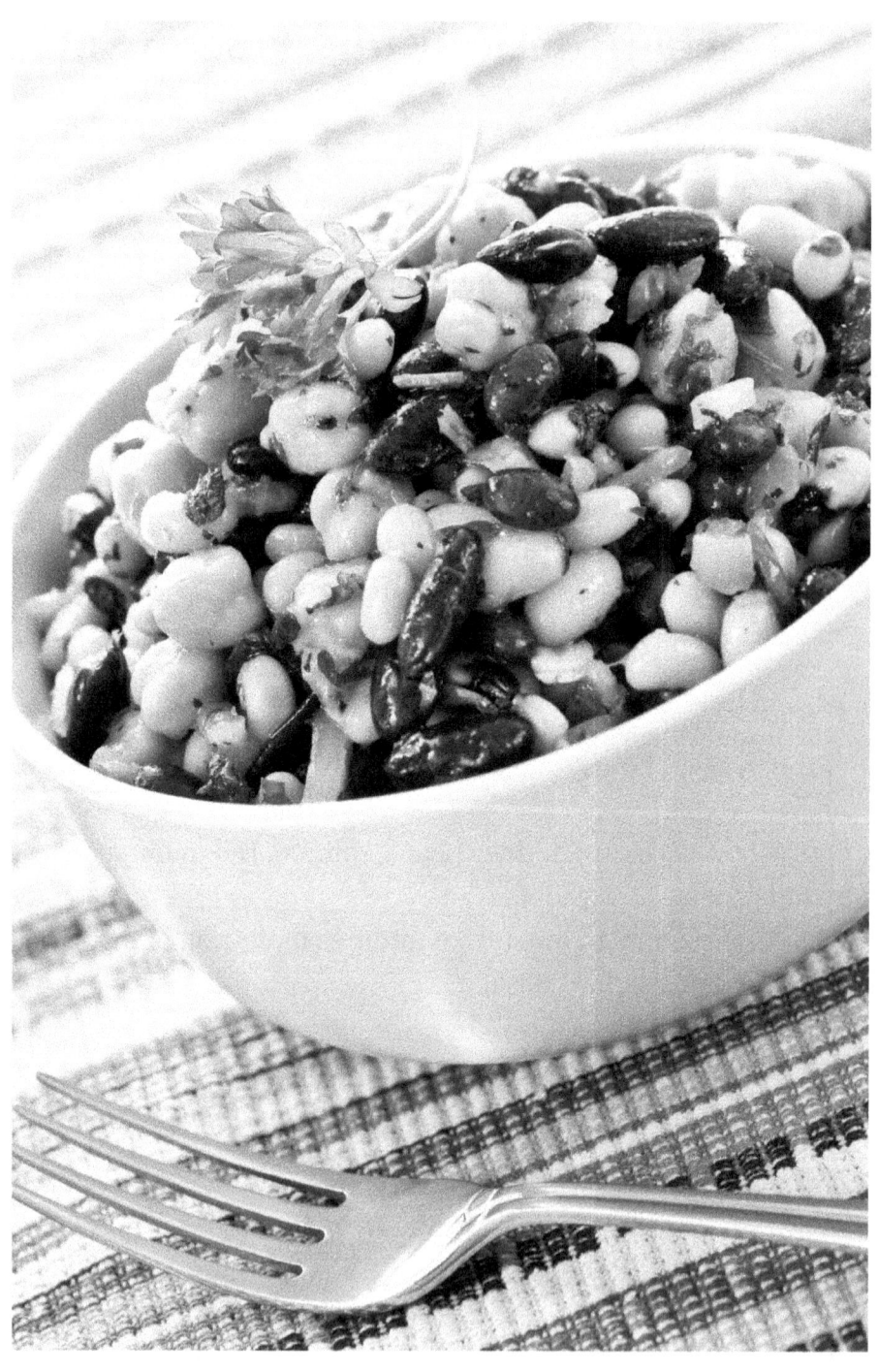

Rice & Currant Salad Mediterranean Style

Servings: 4
Cooking Time: 50 Minutes

Ingredients:
- 1 cup basmati rice
- salt
- 2 1/2 Tablespoons lemon juice
- 1 teaspoon grated orange zest
- 2 Tablespoons fresh orange juice
- 1/4 cup olive oil
- 1/2 teaspoon cinnamon
- Salt and pepper to taste
- 4 chopped green onions
- 1/2 cup dried currants
- 3/4 cup shelled pistachios or almonds
- 1/4 cup chopped fresh parsley

Directions:
1. Place a nonstick pot on medium high fire and add rice. Toast rice until opaque and starts to smell, around 10 minutes.
2. Add 4 quarts of boiling water to pot and 2 tsp salt. Boil until tender, around 8 minutes uncovered.
3. Drain the rice and spread out on a lined cookie sheet to cool completely.
4. In a large salad bowl, whisk well the oil, juices and spices. Add salt and pepper to taste.
5. Add half of the green onions, half of parsley, currants, and nuts.
6. Toss with the cooled rice and let stand for at least 20 minutes.

7. If needed adjust seasoning with pepper and salt.
8. Garnish with remaining parsley and green onions.

Nutrition Info: Calories per serving: 450; Carbs: 50.0g; Protein: 9.0g; Fat: 24.0g

Stuffed Tomatoes With Green Chili

Servings: 6
Cooking Time: 55 Minutes

Ingredients:
- 4 oz Colby-Jack shredded cheese
- ¼ cup water
- 1 cup uncooked quinoa
- 6 large ripe tomatoes
- ¼ tsp freshly ground black pepper
- ¾ tsp ground cumin
- 1 tsp salt, divided
- 1 tbsp fresh lime juice
- 1 tbsp olive oil
- 1 tbsp chopped fresh oregano
- 1 cup chopped onion
- 2 cups fresh corn kernels
- 2 poblano chilies

Directions:
1. Preheat the broiler to high.
2. Slice lengthwise the chilies and press on a baking sheet lined with foil. Broil for 8 minutes. Remove from oven and let cool for 10 minutes. Peel the chilies and chop coarsely and place in medium sized bowl.
3. Place onion and corn in baking sheet and broil for ten minutes. Stir two times while broiling. Remove from oven and mix in with chopped chilies.
4. Add black pepper, cumin, ¼ tsp salt, lime juice, oil and oregano. Mix well.

5. Cut off the tops of tomatoes and set aside. Leave the tomato shell intact as you scoop out the tomato pulp.
6. Drain tomato pulp as you press down with a spoon. Reserve 1 ¼ cups of tomato pulp liquid and discard the rest. Invert the tomato shells on a wire rack for 30 mins and then wipe the insides dry with a paper towel.
7. Season with ½ tsp salt the tomato pulp.
8. On a sieve over a bowl, place quinoa. Add water until it covers quinoa. Rub quinoa grains for 30 seconds together with hands; rinse and drain. Repeat this procedure two times and drain well at the end.
9. In medium saucepan bring to a boil remaining salt, ¼ cup water, quinoa and tomato liquid.
10. Once boiling, reduce heat and simmer for 15 minutes or until liquid is fully absorbed. Remove from heat and fluff quinoa with fork. Transfer and mix well the quinoa with the corn mixture.
11. Spoon ¾ cup of the quinoa-corn mixture into the tomato shells, top with cheese and cover with the tomato top. Bake in a preheated 350oF oven for 15 minutes and then broil high for another 1.5 minutes.

Nutrition Info: Calories per serving: 276; Carbs: 46.3g; Protein: 13.4g; Fat: 4.1g

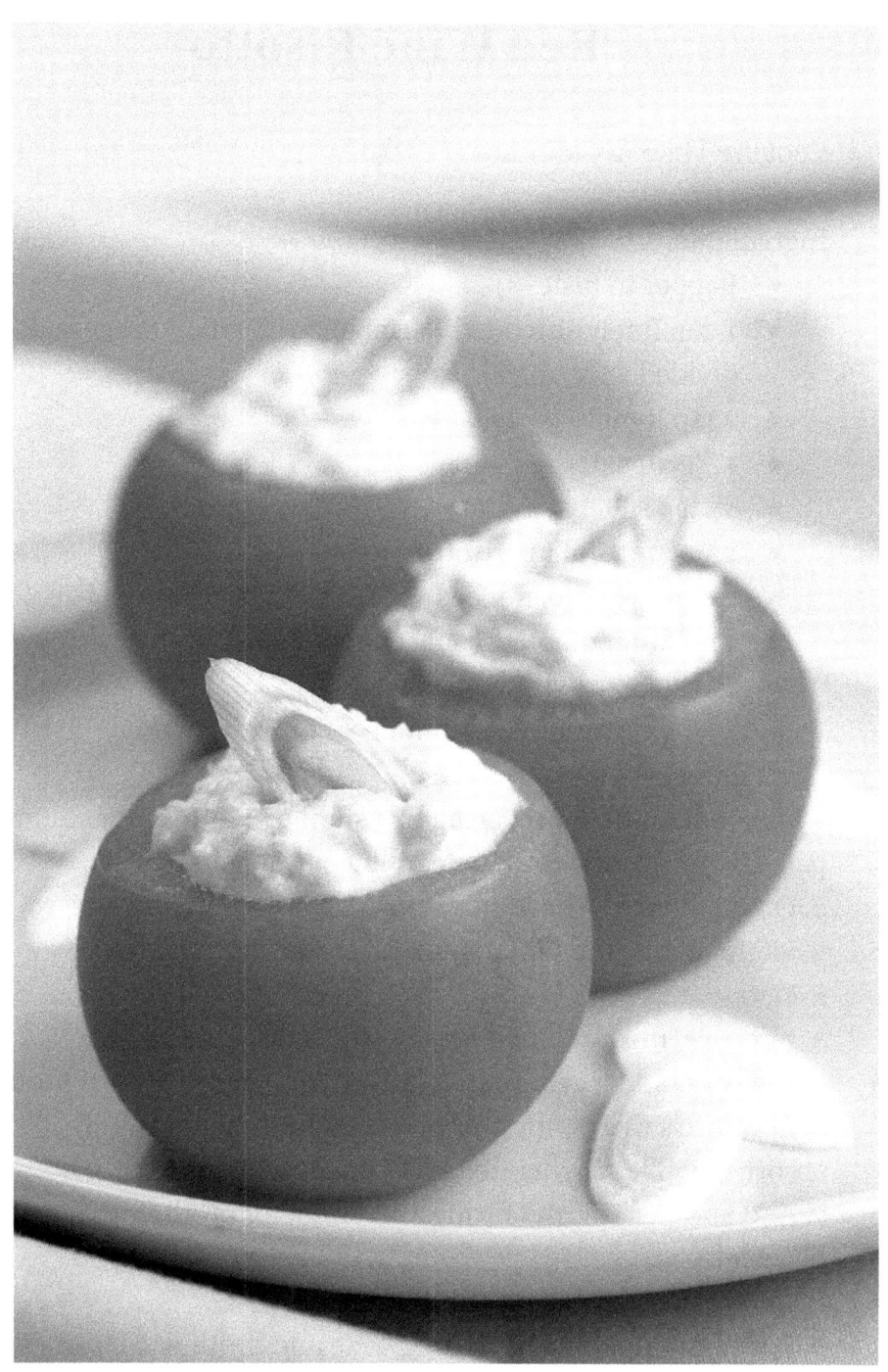

Red Wine Risotto

Servings: 8
Cooking Time: 25 Minutes

Ingredients:
- Pepper to taste
- 1 cup finely shredded Parmigiano-Reggiano cheese, divided
- 2 tsp tomato paste
- 1 ¾ cups dry red wine
- ¼ tsp salt
- 1 ½ cups Italian 'risotto' rice
- 2 cloves garlic, minced
- 1 medium onion, freshly chopped
- 2 tbsp extra-virgin olive oil
- 4 ½ cups reduced sodium beef broth

Directions:
1. On medium high fire, bring to a simmer broth in a medium fry pan. Lower fire so broth is steaming but not simmering.
2. On medium low heat, place a Dutch oven and heat oil.
3. Sauté onions for 5 minutes. Add garlic and cook for 2 minutes.
4. Add rice, mix well, and season with salt.
5. Into rice, add a generous splash of wine and ½ cup of broth.
6. Lower fire to a gentle simmer, cook until liquid is fully absorbed while stirring rice every once in a while.
7. Add another splash of wine and ½ cup of broth. Stirring once in a while.
8. Add tomato paste and stir to mix well.
9. Continue cooking and adding wine and broth until broth is used up.

10. Once done cooking, turn off fire and stir in pepper and ¾ cup cheese.
11. To serve, sprinkle with remaining cheese and enjoy.

Nutrition Info: Calories per Serving: 231; Carbs: 33.9g; Protein: 7.9g; Fat: 5.7g

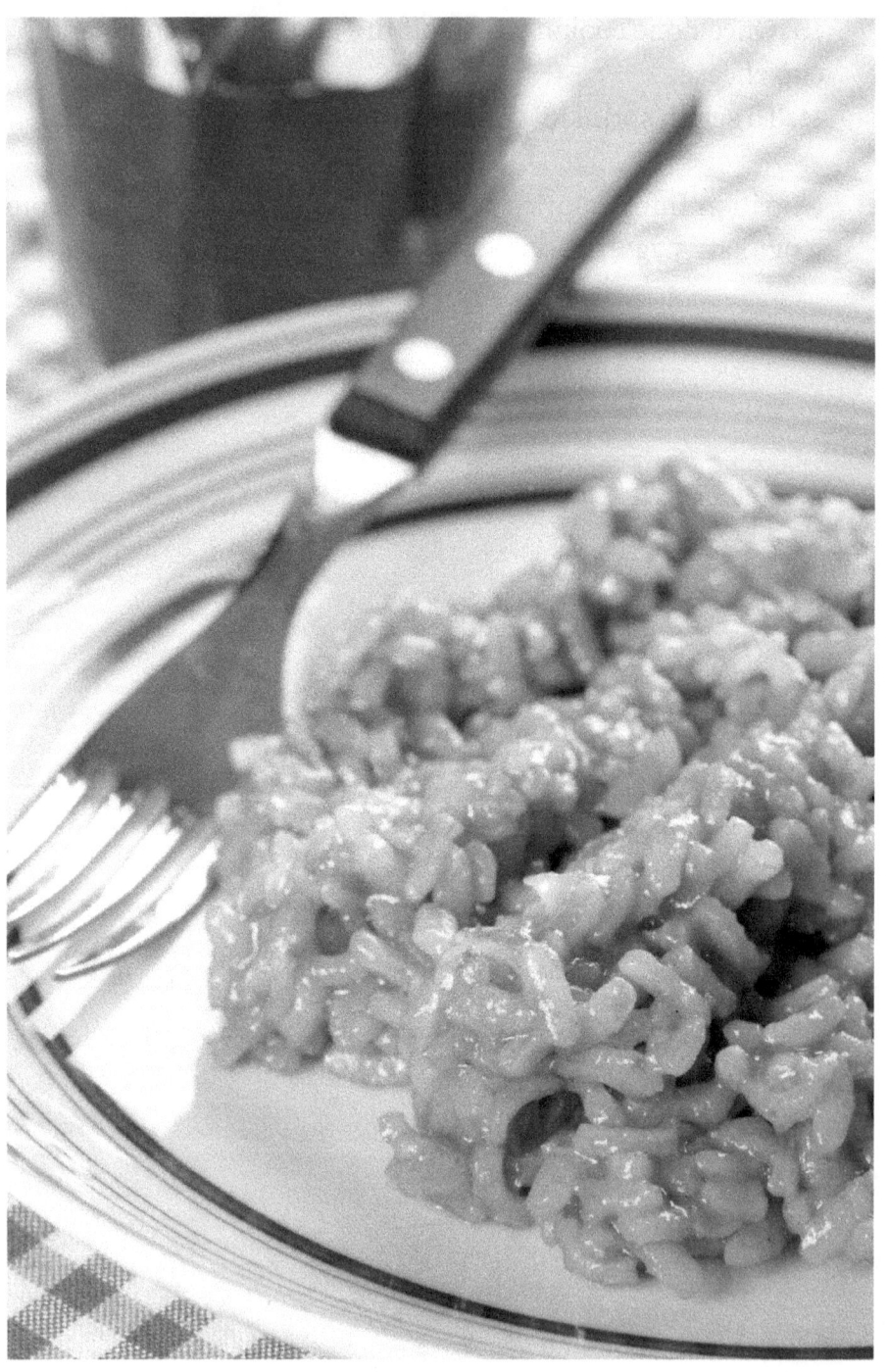

Pasta Parmesan

Servings: 1
Cooking Time: 20 Minutes

Ingredients:
- ¼ cup prepared marinara sauce
- ½ cup cooked whole wheat spaghetti
- 1 oz reduced fat mozzarella cheese, grated
- 1 tbsp olive oil
- 2 tbsp seasoned dry breadcrumbs
- 4 oz skinless chicken breast

Directions:
1. On medium high fire, place an ovenproof skillet and heat oil.
2. Pan fry chicken for 3 to 5 minutes per side or until cooked through.
3. Pour marinara sauce, stir and continue cooking for 3 minutes.
4. Turn off fire, add mozzarella and breadcrumbs on top.
5. Pop into a preheated broiler on high and broil for 10 minutes or until breadcrumbs are browned and mozzarella is melted.
6. Remove from broiler, serve and enjoy.

Nutrition Info: Calories per Serving: 529; Carbs: 34.4g; Protein: 38g; Fat: 26.6g

Orange, Dates And Asparagus On Quinoa Salad

Servings: 8
Cooking Time: 25 Minutes

Ingredients:
- ¼ cup chopped pecans, toasted
- ½ cup white onion, finely chopped
- ½ jalapeno pepper, diced
- ½ lb. asparagus, sliced into 2-inch lengths, steamed and chilled ½ tsp salt
- 1 cup fresh orange sections
- 1 cup uncooked quinoa
- 1 tsp olive oil
- 2 cups water
- 2 tbsp minced red onion
- 5 dates, pitted and chopped
- ¼ tsp freshly ground black pepper
- ¼ tsp salt
- 1 garlic clove, minced
- 1 tbsp extra virgin olive oil
- 2 tbsp chopped fresh mint
- 2 tbsp fresh lemon juice
- Mint sprigs – optional

Directions:
1. On medium high fire, place a large nonstick pan and heat 1 tsp oil.
2. Add white onion and sauté for two minutes.
3. Add quinoa and for 5 minutes sauté it.

4. Add salt and water. Bring to a boil, once boiling, slow fire to a simmer and cook for 15 minutes while covered.
5. Turn off fire and leave for 15 minutes, to let quinoa absorb the remaining water.
6. Transfer quinoa to a large salad bowl. Add jalapeno pepper, asparagus, dates, red onion, pecans and oranges. Toss to combine.
7. Make the dressing by mixing garlic, pepper, salt, olive oil and lemon juice in a small bowl.
8. Pour dressing into quinoa salad along with chopped mint, mix well. 9. If desired, garnish with mint sprigs before serving.

Nutrition Info: Calories per Serving: 265.2; Carbs: 28.3g; Protein: 14.6g; Fat: 10.4g

Tasty Lasagna Rolls

Servings: 6

Cooking Time: 20 Minutes

Ingredients:
- ¼ tsp crushed red pepper
- ¼ tsp salt
- ½ cup shredded mozzarella cheese
- ½ cups parmesan cheese, shredded
- 1 14-oz package tofu, cubed
- 1 25-oz can of low-sodium marinara sauce
- 1 tbsp extra virgin olive oil
- 12 whole wheat lasagna noodles
- 2 tbsp Kalamata olives, chopped
- 3 cloves minced garlic
- 3 cups spinach, chopped

Directions:

1. Put enough water on a large pot and cook the lasagna noodles according to package instructions. Drain, rinse and set aside until ready to use.

2. In a large skillet, sauté garlic over medium heat for 20 seconds. Add the tofu and spinach and cook until the spinach wilts. Transfer this mixture in a bowl and add parmesan olives, salt, red pepper and 2/3 cup of the marinara sauce.

3. In a pan, spread a cup of marinara sauce on the bottom. To make the rolls, place noodle on a surface and spread ¼ cup of the tofu filling. Roll up and place it on the pan with the marinara sauce. Do this procedure until all lasagna noodles are rolled.

4. Place the pan over high heat and bring to a simmer. Reduce the heat to medium and let it cook for three more minutes.

Sprinkle mozzarella cheese and let the cheese melt for two minutes. Serve hot.

Nutrition Info: Calories per Serving: 304; Carbs: 39.2g; Protein: 23g; Fat: 19.2g

Raisins, Nuts And Beef On Hashweh Rice

Servings: 8
Cooking Time: 50 Minutes

Ingredients:
- ½ cup dark raisins, soaked in 2 cups water for an hour
- 1/3 cup slivered almonds, toasted and soaked in 2 cups water overnight 1/3 cup pine nuts, toasted and soaked in 2 cups water overnight ½ cup fresh parsley leaves, roughly chopped
- Pepper and salt to taste
- ¾ tsp ground cinnamon, divided
- ¾ tsp cloves, divided
- 1 tsp garlic powder
- 1 ¾ tsp allspice, divided
- 1 lb. lean ground beef or lean ground lamb
- 1 small red onion, finely chopped
- Olive oil
- 1 ½ cups medium grain rice

Directions:
1. For 15 to 20 minutes, soak rice in cold water. You will know that soaking is enough when you can snap a grain of rice easily between your thumb and index finger. Once soaking is done, drain rice well.
2. Meanwhile, drain pine nuts, almonds and raisins for at least a minute and transfer to one bowl. Set aside.
3. On a heavy cooking pot on medium high fire, heat 1 tbsp olive oil.

4. Once oil is hot, add red onions. Sauté for a minute before adding ground
meat and sauté for another minute.
5. Season ground meat with pepper, salt, ½ tsp ground cinnamon, ½ tsp ground cloves, 1 tsp garlic powder, and 1 ¼ tsp allspice.
6. Sauté ground meat for 10 minutes or until browned and cooked fully. Drain fat.
7. In same pot with cooked ground meat, add rice on top of meat.
8. Season with a bit of pepper and salt. Add remaining cinnamon, ground cloves, and allspice. Do not mix.
9. Add 1 tbsp olive oil and 2 ½ cups of water. Bring to a boil and once boiling, lower fire to a simmer. Cook while covered until liquid is fully absorbed, around 20 to 25 minutes.
10. Turn of fire.
11. To serve, place a large serving platter that fully covers the mouth of the pot. Place platter upside down on mouth of pot, and invert pot. The inside of the pot should now rest on the platter with the rice on bottom of plate and ground meat on top of it.
12. Garnish the top of the meat with raisins, almonds, pine nuts, and parsley.
13. Serve and enjoy.

Nutrition Info: Calories per serving: 357; Carbs: 39.0g; Protein: 16.7g; Fat: 15.9g

Yangchow Chinese Style Fried Rice

Servings: 4
Cooking Time: 20 Minutes

Ingredients:
- 4 cups cold cooked rice
- 1/2 cup peas
- 1 medium yellow onion, diced
- 5 tbsp olive oil
- 4 oz frozen medium shrimp, thawed, shelled, deveined and chopped finely
- 6 oz roast pork
- 3 large eggs
- Salt and freshly ground black pepper
- 1/2 tsp cornstarch

Directions:
1. Combine the salt and ground black pepper and 1/2 tsp cornstarch, coat the shrimp with it. Chop the roasted pork. Beat the eggs and set aside.
2. Stir-fry the shrimp in a wok on high fire with 1 tbsp heated oil until pink, around 3 minutes. Set the shrimp aside and stir fry the roasted pork briefly. Remove both from the pan.
3. In the same pan, stir-fry the onion until soft, Stir the peas and cook until bright green. Remove both from pan.
4. Add 2 tbsp oil in the same pan, add the cooked rice. Stir and separate the individual grains. Add the beaten eggs, toss the rice. Add the roasted pork, shrimp, vegetables and onion. Toss everything together. Season with salt and pepper to taste.

Nutrition Info: Calories per serving: 556; Carbs: 60.2g; Protein: 20.2g; Fat: 25.2g

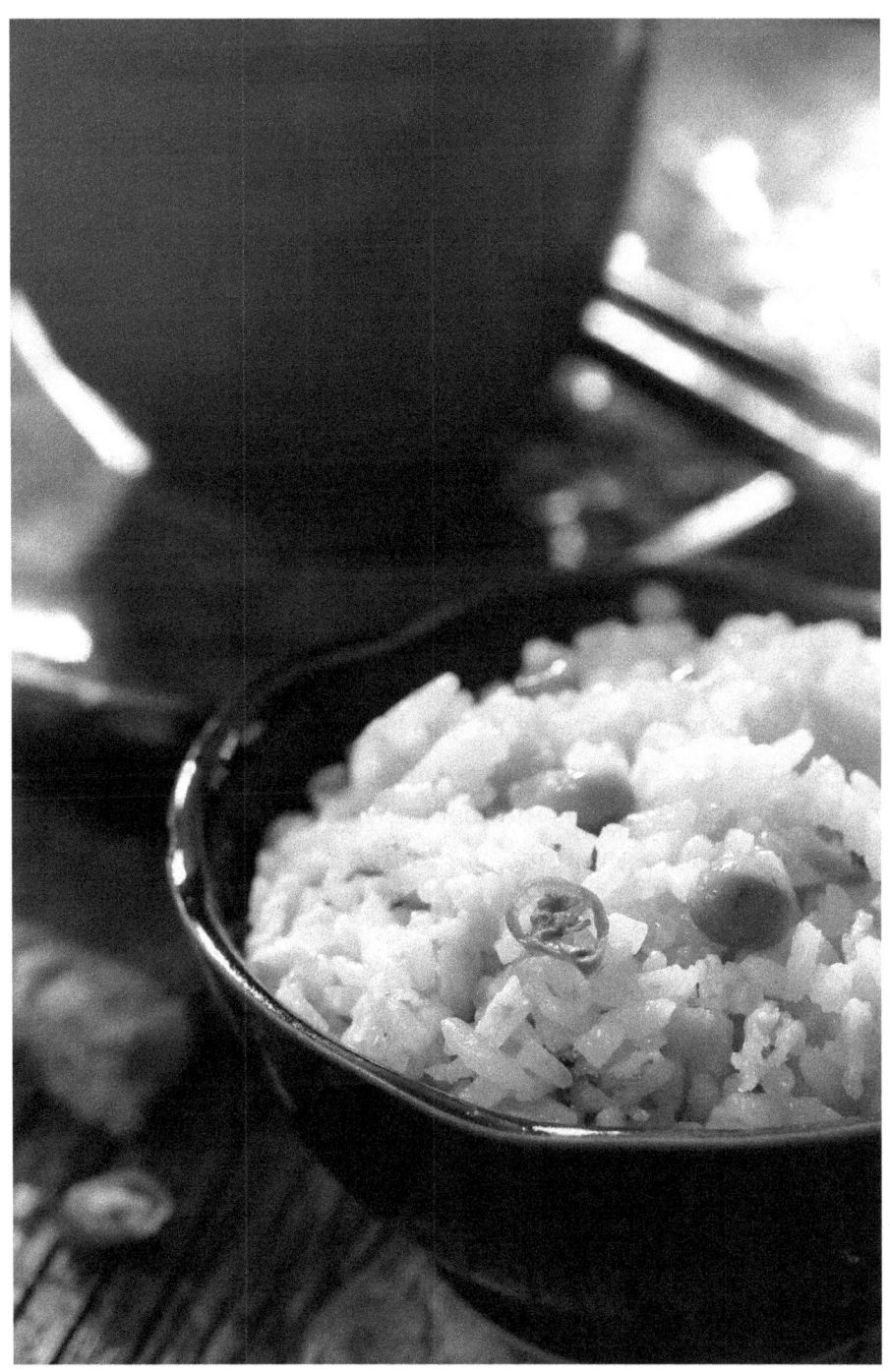

Cinnamon Quinoa Bars

Servings: 4
Cooking Time: 30 Minutes

Ingredients:
- 2 ½ cups cooked quinoa
- 4 large eggs
- 1/3 cup unsweetened almond milk
- 1/3 cup pure maple syrup
- Seeds from ½ whole vanilla bean pod or 1 tbsp vanilla extract 1 ½ tbsp cinnamon
- 1/4 tsp salt

Directions:
1. Preheat oven to 375oF.
2. Combine all ingredients into large bowl and mix well.
3. In an 8 x 8 Baking pan, cover with parchment paper.
4. Pour batter evenly into baking dish.
5. Bake for 25-30 minutes or until it has set. It should not wiggle when you lightly shake the pan because the eggs are fully cooked.
6. Remove as quickly as possible from pan and parchment paper onto cooling rack.
7. Cut into 4 pieces.
8. Enjoy on its own, with a small spread of almond or nut butter or wait until it cools to enjoy the next morning.

Nutrition Info: Calories per serving: 285; Carbs: 46.2g; Protein: 8.5g; Fat: 7.4g

Cucumber Olive Rice

Servings: 8
Cooking Time: 10 Minutes
Ingredients:
- 2 cups rice, rinsed
- 1/2 cup olives, pitted
- 1 cup cucumber, chopped
- 1 tbsp red wine vinegar
- 1 tsp lemon zest, grated
- 1 tbsp fresh lemon juice
- 2 tbsp olive oil
- 2 cups vegetable broth
- 1/2 tsp dried oregano
- 1 red bell pepper, chopped
- 1/2 cup onion, chopped
- 1 tbsp olive oil
- Pepper
- Salt

Directions:
1. Add oil into the inner pot of instant pot and set the pot on sauté mode.
2. Add onion and sauté for 3 minutes.
3. Add bell pepper and oregano and sauté for 1 minute.
4. Add rice and broth and stir well.
5. Seal pot with lid and cook on high for 6 minutes.
6. Once done, allow to release pressure naturally for 10 minutes then release remaining using quick release. Remove lid.
7. Add remaining ingredients and stir everything well to mix. 8. Serve immediately and enjoy it.

Nutrition Info: Calories 229 Fat 5.1 g Carbohydrates 40.2 g Sugar 1.6 g Protein 4.9 g Cholesterol 0 mg

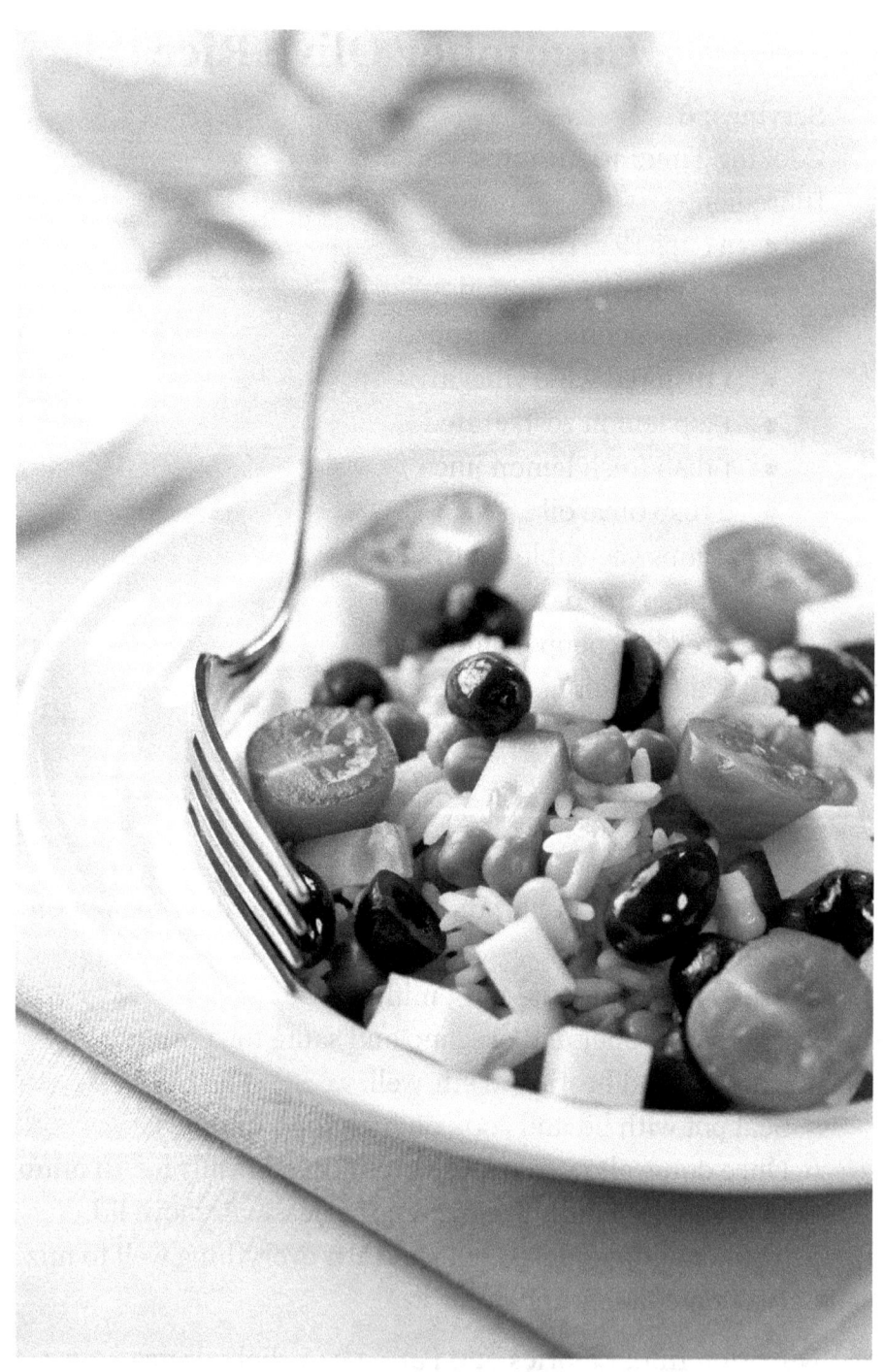

Desserts

Soothing Red Smoothie

Servings: 2
Cooking Time: 3 Minutes

Ingredients:
- 4 plums, pitted
- ¼ cup raspberry
- ¼ cup blueberry
- 1 tablespoon lemon juice
- 1 tablespoon linseed oil

Directions:
1. Place all Ingredients: in a blender.
2. Blend until smooth.
3. Pour in a glass container and allow to chill in the fridge for at least 30 minutes.

Nutrition Info: Calories per serving: 201; Carbs: 36.4g; Protein: 0.8g; Fat: 7.1g

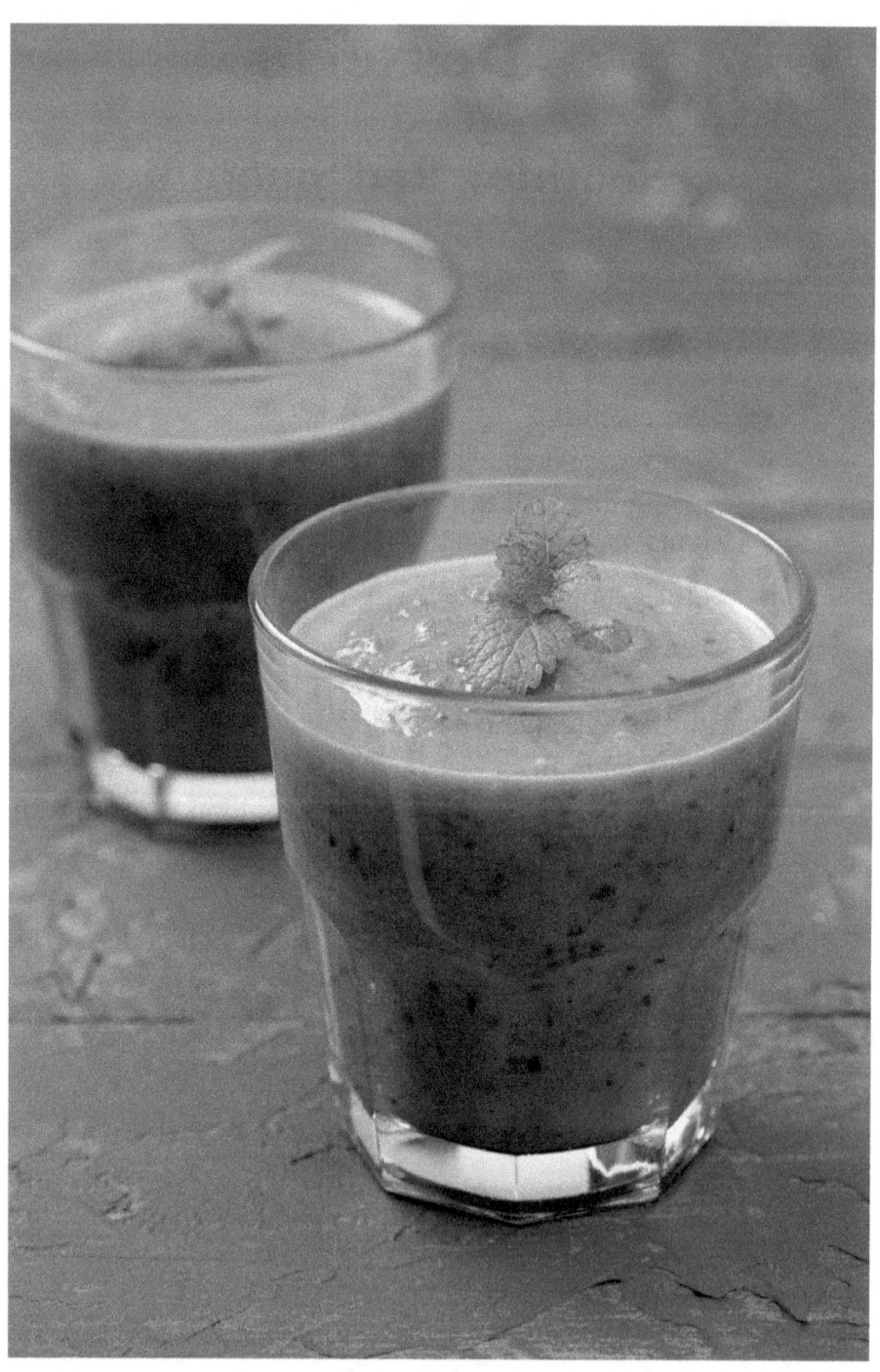

Minty Orange Greek Yogurt

Servings: 1
Cooking Time: 5 Minutes

Ingredients:
- 6 tablespoons Greek yogurt, fat-free
- 4 fresh mint leaves, thinly sliced
- 1 large orange, peeled, quartered, and then sliced crosswise
- 1 1/2 teaspoons honey

Directions:
1. Stir together the honey and the yogurt.
2. Place the orange slices into a dessert glass. Spoon the honeyed yogurt over the orange slices in the glass and scatter the mint on top of the yogurt.

Nutrition Info:Per Serving:171 cal., 34 g total carbs, 5 g fiber, and 11 g protein.

Yogurt Mousse With Sour Cherry Sauce

Servings: 6
Cooking Time: 1 Hour

Ingredients:
- 1 ½ cups Greek yogurt
- 1 teaspoon vanilla extract
- 4 tablespoons honey
- 1 ½ cups heavy cream, whipped
- 2 cups sour cherries
- ¼ cup white sugar
- 1 cinnamon stick

Directions:
1. Combine the yogurt with vanilla and honey in a bowl.
2. Fold in the whipped cream then spoon the mousse into serving glasses and refrigerate.
3. For the sauce, combine the cherries, sugar and cinnamon in a saucepan. Allow to rest for 10 minutes then cook on low heat for 10 minutes.
4. Cool the sauce down then spoon it over the mousse.
5. Serve it right away.

Nutrition Info: Per Serving:Calories:245 Fat:12.1g Protein:5.8g Carbohydrates:29.7g

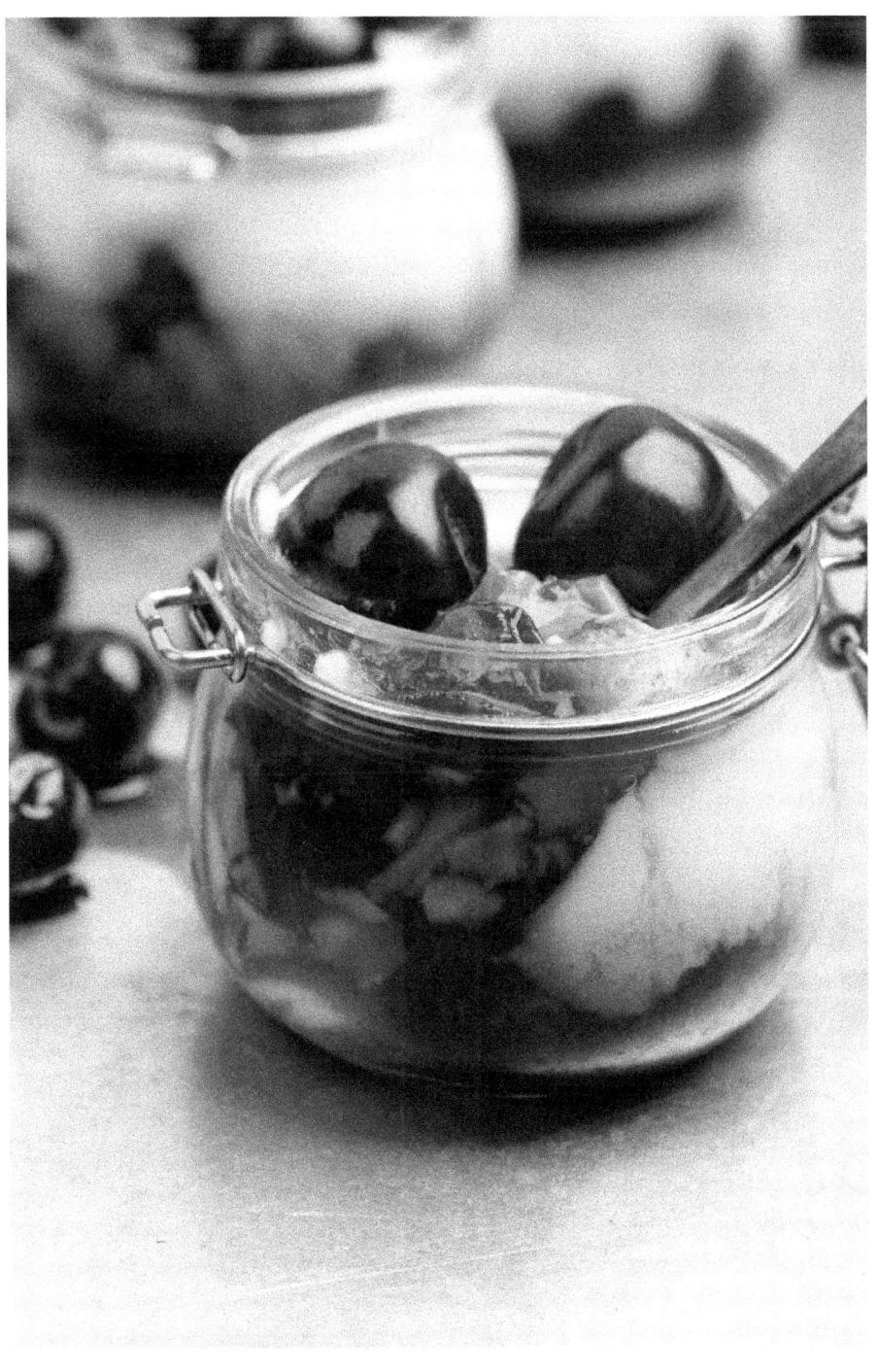

Vanilla Apple Pie

Servings: 8
Cooking Time: 50 Minutes

Ingredients:
- 3 apples, sliced
- ½ teaspoon ground cinnamon
- 1 teaspoon vanilla extract
- 1 tablespoon Erythritol
- 7 oz yeast roll dough
- 1 egg, beaten

Directions:
1. Roll up the dough and cut it on 2 parts.
2. Line the springform pan with baking paper.
3. Place the first dough part in the springform pan.
4. Then arrange the apples over the dough and sprinkle it with Erythritol, vanilla extract, and ground cinnamon.
5. Then cover the apples with remaining dough and secure the edges of the pie with the help of the fork.
6. Make the small cuts in the surface of the pie.
7. Brush the pie with beaten egg and bake it for 50 minutes at 375F. 8. Cool the cooked pie well and then remove from the springform pan. 9. Cut it on the servings.

Nutrition Info:Per Serving:calories 139, fat 3.6, fiber 3.1, carbs 26.1, protein 2.8

Spinach Pancake Cake

Servings: 6
Cooking Time: 15 Minutes

Ingredients:
- 1 cup heavy cream
- ¼ cup Erythritol
- 1 cup fresh spinach, chopped
- ½ cup skim milk
- 1 teaspoon vanilla extract
- 1 cup all-purpose flour
- ½ cup of rice flour
- 1 teaspoon baking powder
- 1 teaspoon olive oil
- 1 egg, beaten
- ¼ teaspoon ground clove
- 1 teaspoon butter

Directions:
1. Blend the spinach until you get puree mixture.
2. After this, add skim milk, vanilla extract, all-purpose flour, and rice flour.
3. Add baking powder, egg, and ground clove.
4. Blend the ingredients until you get a smooth and thick batter.
5. Then add olive oil and pulse the batter for 30 seconds more.
6. Heat up butter in the skillet.
7. Ladle 1 ladle of the crepe batter in the skillet and flatten it in the shape of crepe.
8. Cook it for 1.5 minutes from one side and them flip into another side and cook for 20 seconds more.
9. Place the cooked crepe in the plate.

10. Repeat the same steps will all crepe batter.
11. Make the cake filling: whip the heavy cream with Erythritol.
12. Spread every crepe with sweet whipped cream.
13. Store the cake in the fridge for up to 2 days.

Nutrition Info:Per Serving:calories 228, fat 10, fiber 1, carbs 38.8, protein 5.1

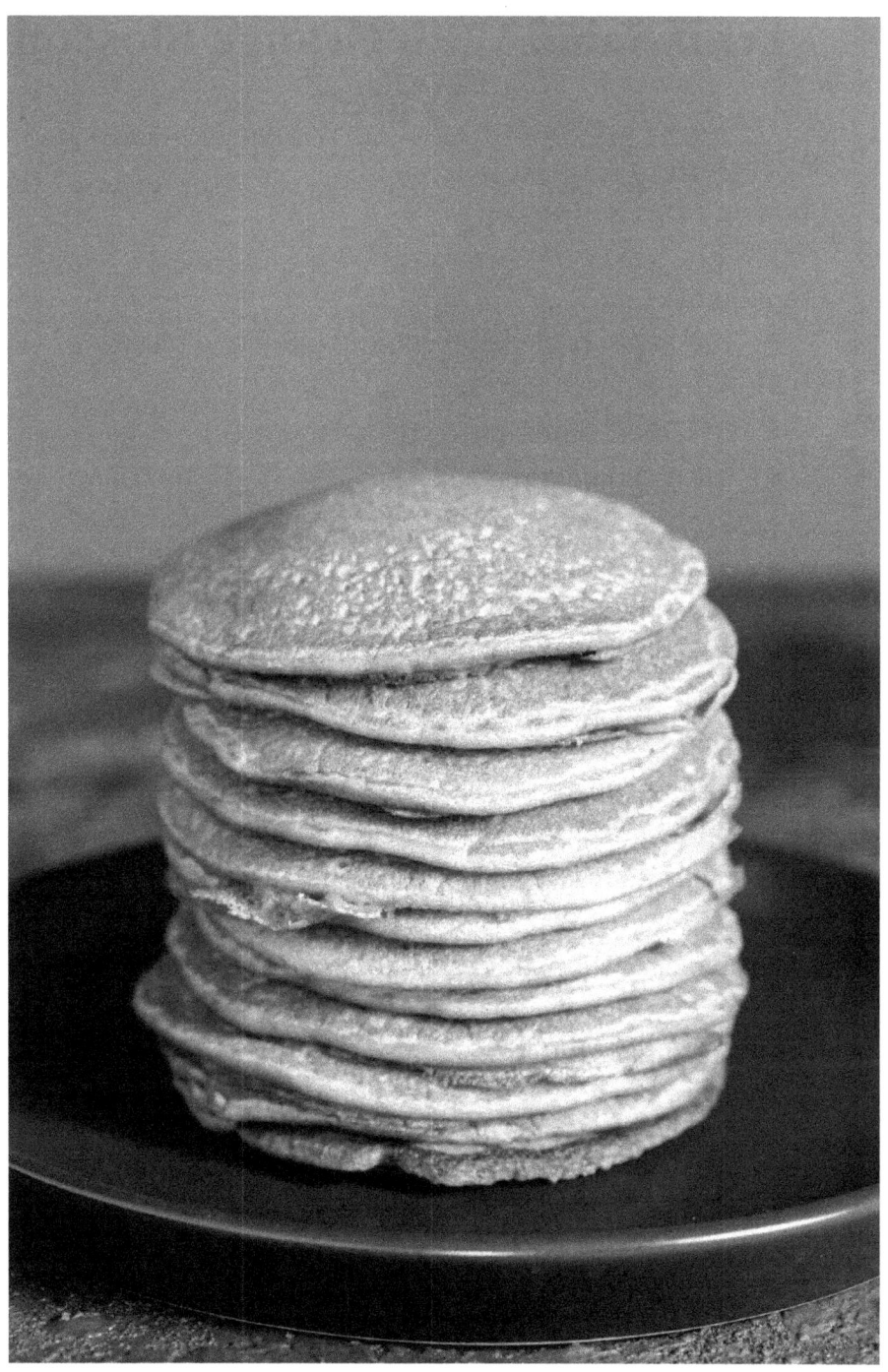

Fruit Salad With Orange Blossom Water

Servings: 8
Cooking Time: 3 Minutes

Ingredients:
- 4 oranges, peeled and cut into bite-sized pieces
- 8 dried figs, quartered
- 2 Medjool dates, pitted then chopped
- ½ cup pomegranate seeds
- 2 tablespoons honey
- 2 tablespoons orange blossom water
- 2 bananas, peeled and sliced
- ¼ cup pistachio nuts, shelled and chopped

Directions:
1. In a large mixing bowl, toss in all the ingredients except for the pistachio nuts.
2. Let the fruits rest in the fridge for at least 8 hours before serving.
3. Garnish with chopped pistachios before serving.

Nutrition Info: Calories per serving: 185; Carbs: 43g; Protein: 3g; Fat: 2g

Blueberry Frozen Yogurt

Servings: 6
Cooking Time: 30 Minutes

Ingredients:
- 1-pint blueberries, fresh
- 2/3 cup honey
- 1 small lemon, juiced and zested
- 2 cups yogurt, chilled

Directions:
1. In a saucepan, combine the blueberries, honey, lemon juice, and zest.
2. Heat over medium heat and allow to simmer for 15 minutes while stirring constantly.
3. Once the liquid has reduced, transfer the fruits in a bowl and allow to cool in the fridge for another 15 minutes.
4. Once chilled, mix together with the chilled yogurt.

Nutrition Info: Calories per serving: 233; Carbs:52.2 g; Protein:3.5 g; Fat: 2.9g

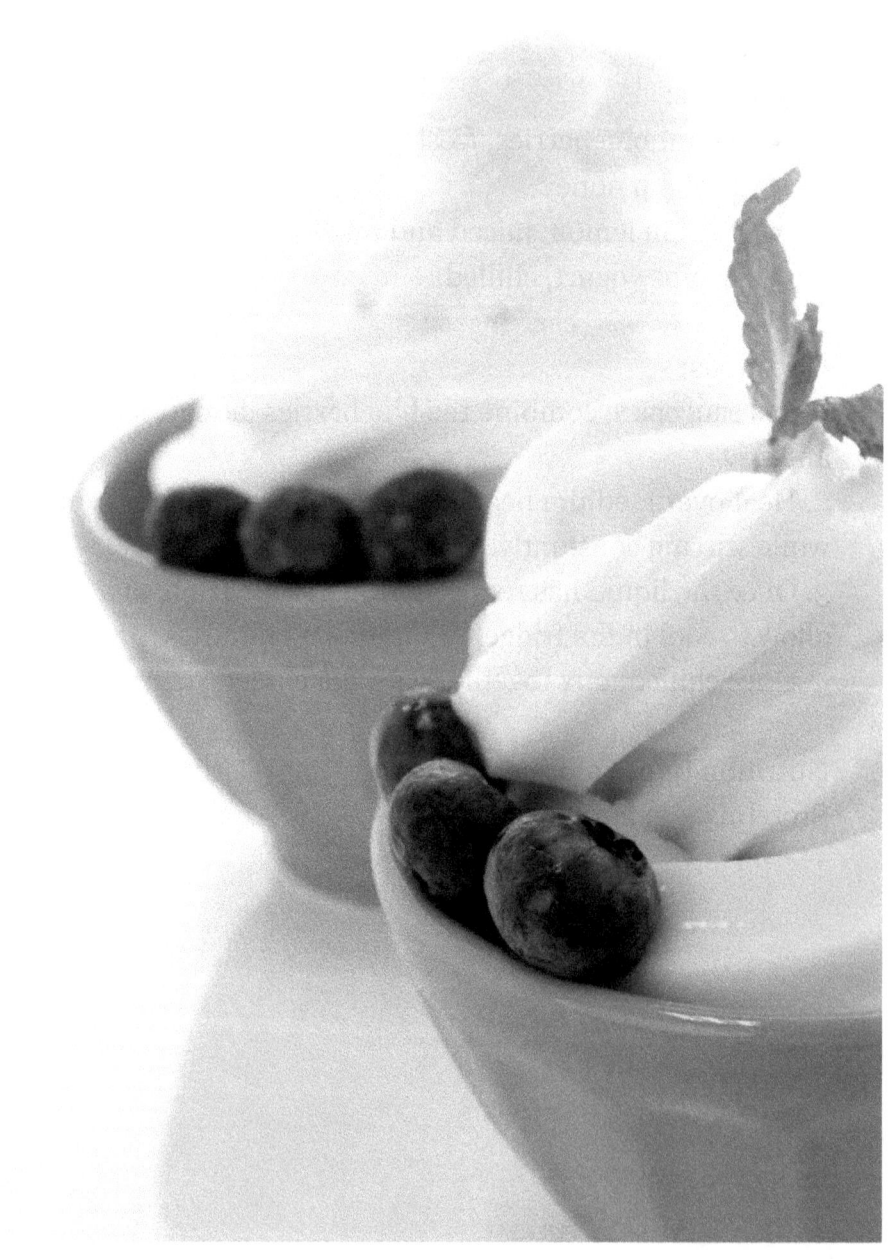

Apple Pear Compote

Servings: 6
Cooking Time: 45 Minutes

Ingredients:
- 4 apples, cored and cubed
- 2 pears, cored and cubed
- 1 cinnamon stick
- 1 star anise
- 2 whole cloves
- 1 orange peel
- 4 cups water
- 2 tablespoons lemon juice

Directions:
1. Combine all the ingredients in a saucepan.
2. Place over low heat and cook for 25 minutes.
3. Serve the compote chilled.

Nutrition Info: Per Serving:Calories:110 Fat:0.5g Protein:0.8g Carbohydrates:28.6g

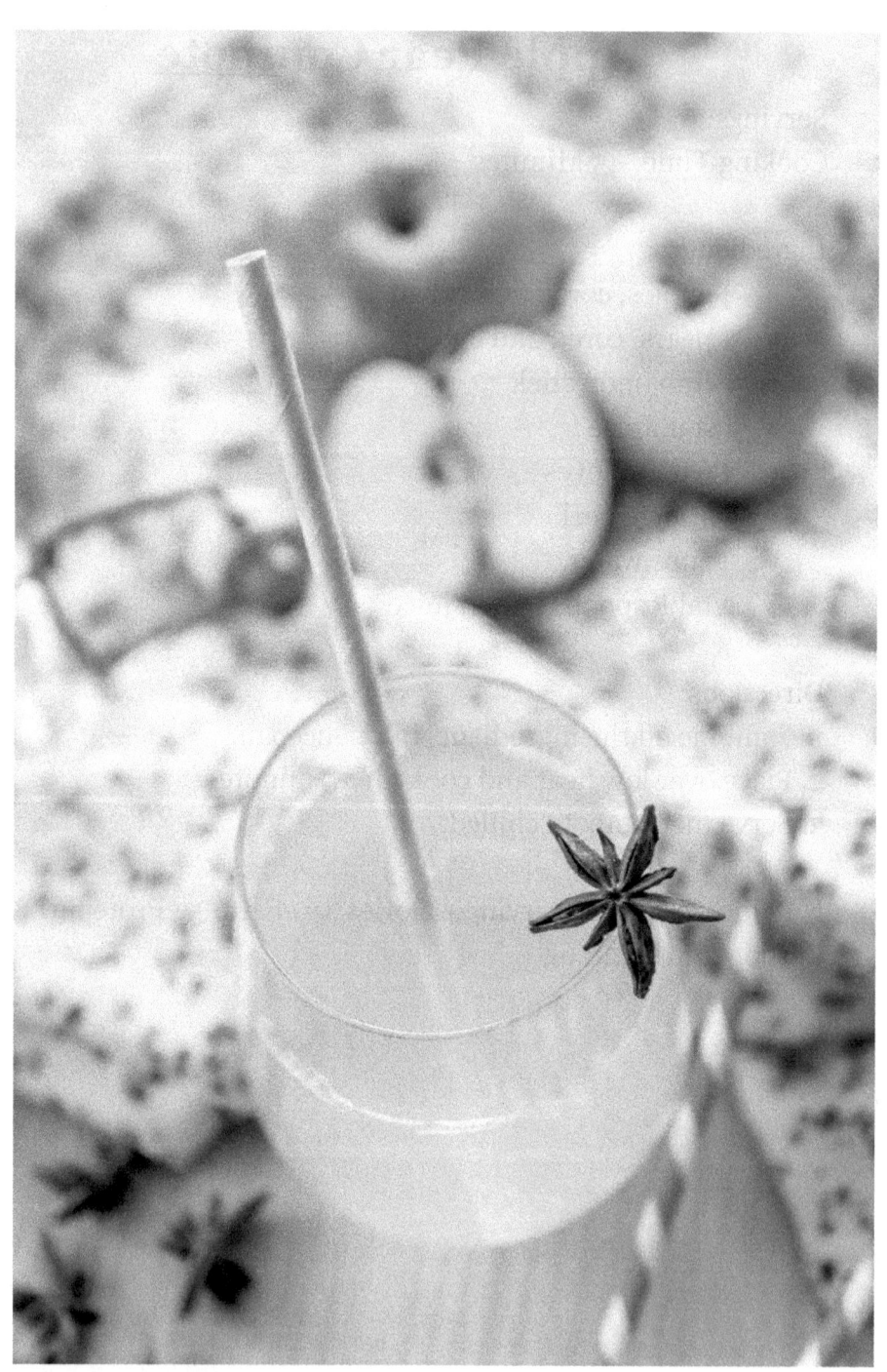

Cream Cheese Cake

Servings: 2
Cooking Time: 60 Minutes

Ingredients:
- 2 teaspoons cream cheese
- 1 cup Erythritol
- 2 egg whites
- ½ teaspoon lemon juice
- ½ teaspoon vanilla extract
- 2 strawberries, sliced

Directions:
1. Whisk the egg whites until you get soft peaks.
2. Keep whisking and gradually add Erythritol and lemon juice.
3. Whisk the egg whites till you get strong peak mass.
4. After this, mix up together cream cheese and vanilla extract.
5. Line the baking tray with baking paper.
6. With the help of the spoon make egg white nests in the tray.
7. Bake the egg white nests for 60 minutes at 205F.
8. When the "nests' are cooked, fill them with vanilla cream cheese and top with sliced strawberries.

Nutrition Info:Per Serving:calories 36, fat 1.3, fiber 0.3, carbs 121.4, protein 3.9

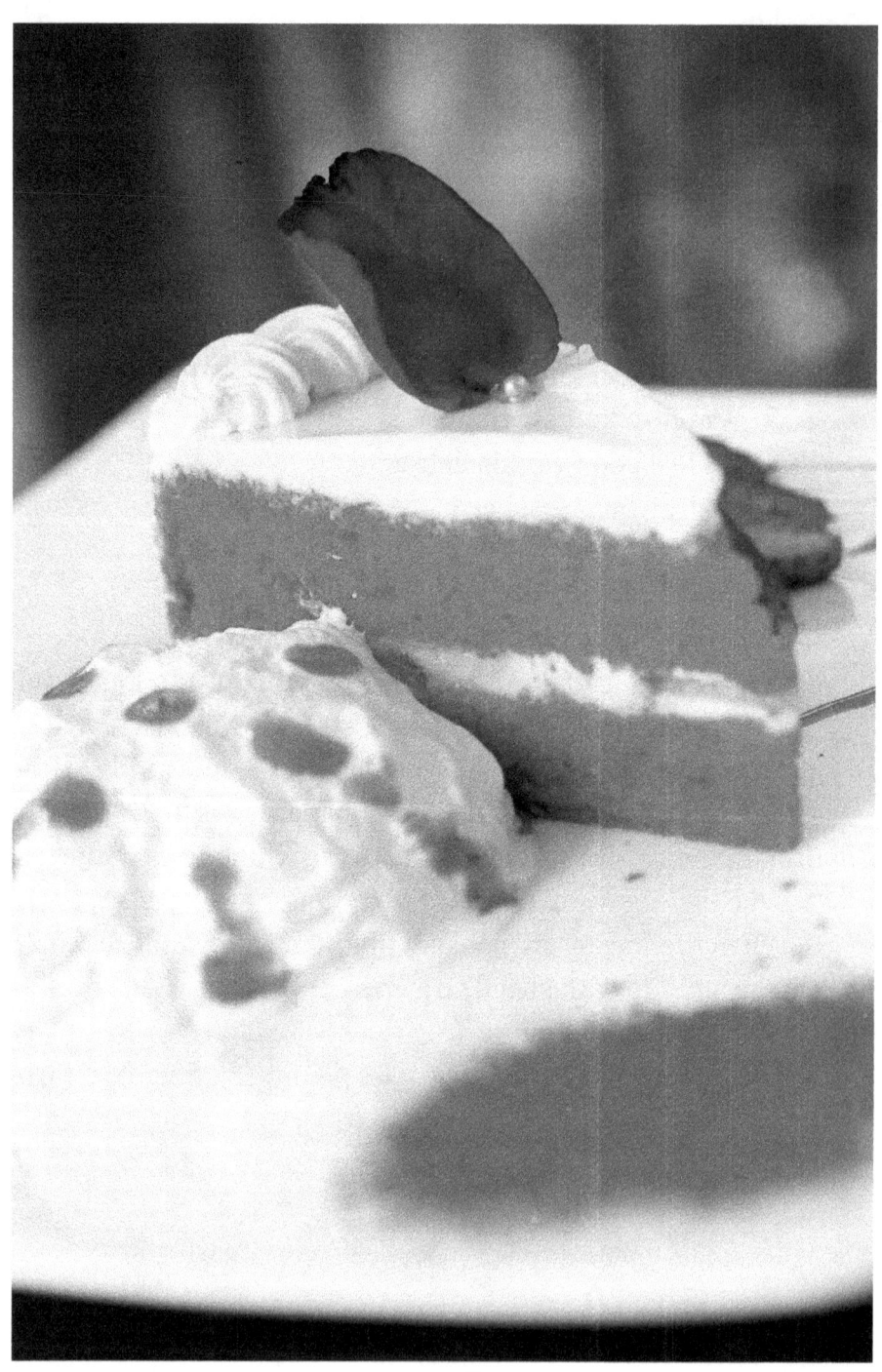

Nutmeg Lemon Pudding

Servings: 6
Cooking Time: 20 Minutes
Ingredients:
- 2 tablespoons lemon marmalade
- 4 eggs, whisked
- 2 tablespoons stevia
- 3 cups almond milk
- 4 allspice berries, crushed
- ¼ teaspoon nutmeg, grated

Directions:
1. In a bowl, mix the lemon marmalade with the eggs and the other ingredients and whisk well.
2. Divide the mix into ramekins, introduce in the oven and bake at 350 degrees F for 20 minutes.
3. Serve cold.

Nutrition Info: calories 220, fat 6.6, fiber 3.4, carbs 12.4, protein 3.4

Yogurt Panna Cotta With Fresh Berries

Servings: 6
Cooking Time: 1 Hour

Ingredients:
- 2 cups Greek yogurt
- 1 cup milk
- 1 cup heavy cream
- 2 teaspoons gelatin powder
- 4 tablespoons cold water
- 4 tablespoons honey
- 1 teaspoon vanilla extract
- 1 teaspoon lemon zest
- 1 pinch salt
- 2 cups mixed berries for serving

Directions:
1. Combine the milk and cream in a saucepan and heat them up.
2. Bloom the gelatin in cold water for 10 minutes.
3. Remove the milk off heat and stir in the gelatin until dissolved.
4. Add the vanilla, lemon zest and salt and allow to cool down.
5. Stir in the yogurt then pour the mixture into serving glasses.
6. When set, top with fresh berries and serve.

Nutrition Info: Per Serving:Calories:219 Fat:9.7g Protein:10.8g Carbohydrates:22.6g

Flourless Chocolate Cake

Servings: 8
Cooking Time: 1 Hour

Ingredients:
- 8 oz. dark chocolate, chopped
- 4 oz. butter, cubed
- 6 eggs, separated
- 1 teaspoon vanilla extract
- 1 pinch salt
- 4 tablespoons white sugar
- Berries for serving

Directions:
1. Combine the chocolate and butter in a heatproof bowl and melt them together until smooth.
2. When smooth, remove off heat and place aside.
3. Separate the eggs.
4. Mix the egg yolks with the chocolate mixture.
5. Whip the egg whites with a pinch of salt until puffed up. Add the sugar and mix for a few more minutes until glossy and stiff.
6. Fold the meringue into the chocolate mixture then pour the batter in a 9- inch round cake pan lined with baking paper.
7. Bake in the preheated oven at 350F for 25 minutes.
8. Serve the cake chilled.

Nutrition Info: Per Serving:Calories:324 Fat:23.2g Protein:6.4g Carbohydrates:23.2g

Notes

www.ingramcontent.com/pod-product-compliance
Lightning Source LLC
Chambersburg PA
CBHW070723030426
42336CB00013B/1904